THE MURDERS AT BULLENHUSER DAMM

The SS Doctor and the Children

Günther Schwarberg

translated by
ERNA BABER ROSENFELD

with
ALVIN H. ROSENFELD

INDIANA UNIVERSITY PRESS • BLOOMINGTON

Published in German as *Der SS-Arzt und die Kinder: Bericht über den Mord vom Bullenhuser Damm*

Manufactured in the United States of America

Library of Congress Cataloging in Publication Data
Schwarberg, Günther.
   The murders at Bullenhuser Damm.

   Translation of: Der SS-Arzt und die Kinder.
   1. World War, 1939–1945—Atrocities. 2. Human experimentation in medicine—Germany—History—20th century. 3. World War, 1939–1945—Children. 4. World War, 1935–1945—Jews. 5. Physicians—Germany. 6. War criminals—Germany. I. Title.
D804.G4S3313   1984   940.54'05   83-48174
ISBN 0-253-15481-2
1 2 3 4 5 88 87 86 85 84

Dedicated to
Irvin Frank, founding chairman of ZACHOR,
the Holocaust Resource Center of the
National Jewish Resource Center, whose
life is his witness that the only way to
respond to the Holocaust is with memory,
love, integrity, and justice,
and to
Frank and May Lipschutz for generously
underwriting the translation of this book

The English translation is
dedicated by May Morgenstern Lipschutz
to Jacqueline Morgenstern,
"a little girl with whom I wanted
to play."

PREFACE

We hear too much about "Holocaust" these days, too little about criminals and their crimes. The present book helps to correct that perspective, for in writing it Günther Schwarberg went in relentless pursuit of some of the Nazi murderers—and found them. Family men, physicians, farmers, former tradesmen, and laborers, these SS officers and concentration camp guards comprised a fair cross section of German society at the time of the Second World War. The reader will find them presented here by name, background, SS-rank, wartime career—and alibi. It is not a pretty picture, and not an easy one for a German author to draw, but as it emerges in these pages it is clear that this is a story we need to know and will not soon be able to forget.

Schwarberg has found many of the victims of these men as well, and their names are also set forth here. In some cases the author was able to reconstruct their family backgrounds and something of their earlier years, but since none was to be given the chance to live beyond the age of twelve, there is not a great deal that can be said about the murdered Jewish children. The fact that we know more about their deaths than about their lives adds to the pathos of their story and helps to account for the mingled feelings of outrage and loss one has in reading it.

The outrage is prompted in large part by what we come to learn about the deeds of the SS and also in no small measure by what we learn of their fate in the postwar period. Some of the SS were brought to trial by the Allied Powers, sentenced, and executed; others managed to evade justice for shorter or longer periods of time; and still others, including some of the worst, were able to take advantage of a lax and weary German judiciary and escape a proper trial altogether. Such people are alive and free today—not always hiding under assumed names in distant lands but often conducting their affairs as normal burghers in the same country where, only a generation ago, they were directly implicated in the killing of vast numbers of people in Hitler's camps.

Once more Schwarberg names names, cites specific crimes, presents detailed observations on what passed as "war-crimes trials," and reveals just how compromised and uncaring members of the German legislature and legal system have been in some instances in handling such cases. This part of Schwarberg's story is more than distressing, for it shows the unwillingness of important segments of postwar German society to come to honest terms with the Nazi past. One wonders, in reading about these trials, just how extensive and effective the so-called denazification program actually was. Everyone knows of Nuremberg and the sentencing of some of the major figures, but what of the countless numbers of others who aided them and without whom the Nazi murder machine would not have run at all? What happened to these people after the war?

Schwarberg describes some of them for us—Kurt Heissmeyer, Arnold Strippel—and in offering vivid case histories of their crimes and the lives they were able to lead afterwards keeps alive this large and disturbing question. It is not the author's intention to present a comprehensive study of the postwar German judiciary or to examine in exhaustive detail the success or failure of the efforts that have or have not been made to identify and bring to justice other former Nazi war criminals. Rather, he has traced the development of a single case—one involving Nazi medical experiments on Jewish children—from its earliest inception, through its torturous culmination, to its sometimes discouraging aftermath before the German courts. What he has discovered forces one to ponder all over again the perplexing phenomenon of highly educated people unwilling or unable to restrain themselves from engaging in the lowest and most revolting kinds of human conduct.

If there are lessons to be learned from this story they have to do with the criminal side of certain kinds of professional ambition and the immoral side of some of the professional disciplines as they have evolved in the modern Western countries. The unsettling fact is that in complex societies one needs but cannot afford to place the entirety of one's trust in people of high professional attainment—people like Dr. Heissmeyer, who said he saw "no difference between guinea pigs and Jewish children" and quite methodically set out to treat the latter as if they were laboratory test animals; or people like Chief Prosecutor Dr. Helmut Münzberg, whom Schwarberg quotes as saying that, while it is true that these children were destroyed, they otherwise "did not suffer *unduly* before they died" and "no further harm was done to them." Once encountered, such sentences are as unforgettable as they are inexplicable. Yet a physician spoke the first, a jurist the second. They will haunt us for a long time to come, these sentences, as will the memories of the Jewish children who fell victim to a social order that produced killers of the kind to be found in the pages of this book.

The book ends with a list of twenty names, the names of the Jewish children who were made to serve as Dr. Heissmeyer's guinea pigs. The ages of the children are given along with their nationalities. In translating this page from the original German edition we felt obliged to make one grammatically small but historically crucial change; namely, we altered the proper nouns ("*Pole,*" "*Niederländer,*" "*Franzose,*" "*Italiener,*" etc.) to versions of these same nouns preceded by the simple preposition "from" ("from Poland," "from Holland," "from France," "from Italy," etc.). To do otherwise might have suggested that the children were murdered *as* Poles, Dutchmen, Frenchmen, Italians; in fact, they were murdered as Jews and only because they were Jews. The plaque originally placed in the Bullenhuser Damm School in Hamburg where they were killed did not say so. Rather, in its somewhat abstract phrasing it commemorated the "twenty *foreign* children" who were murdered on the night of April 20–21, 1945, and went on to beseech everyone to "remember the victims with love" and "to learn to respect man and all human life." The sentiment may have been noble, but it was far too vaguely expressed to encourage true remembrance of what in fact took place in that school in the spring of 1945. For unless and until the children could be acknowledged as young Jews they would remain forever "foreign" and hence still beyond the reach of the very people who need to see their lives and their deaths in intimate historical perspective.

It was precisely this kind of recognition that was needed and in fact came about following the publication of Günther Schwarberg's book. The original plaque with its vague wording has been replaced by a newer, more detailed one, specifying the Jewish identity of the murdered children and also listing the others put to death with them. In addition, a plaque now affixed to the outside of the school calls attention to the fact that the building had served as an auxiliary camp of Neuengamme concentration camp toward the end of the war, and it, too, specifies the nature of the crimes committed there on the evening of April 20, 1945. Still another plaque on the building's exterior is inscribed with the name of Janusz Korczak, the Polish-Jewish physician and writer murdered in Treblinka with a group of Jewish orphans he had attended and tried to protect, and this plaque declares that the Bullenhuser Damm School has been renamed the "Janusz-Korczak Schule." Two rooms in the basement house photographs of the children and documents that describe what happened to them and are open to visits as a museum on a daily basis. Memorial services take place annually at the site on April 20, and a rose garden has been set aside behind the school building as still one more act of commemoration. It is supervised by the Society for the Children of Bullenhuser Damm, a group dedicated to keeping alive the memory of the murdered children.

There remains the question of Arnold Strippel, the SS officer implicated in these crimes. He remains a free citizen of West Germany, lives a comfortable life outside of Frankfurt, and as of this writing does not seem to be in danger of imminent prosecution. As far back as 1967 survivors of Neuengamme sought to open an investigation into Strippel's role in the murders at Bullenhuser Damm, but they proved unsuccessful. More recently, an association of Jews from France, consisting of members of the families of the children together with surviving relatives of other Jews deported from France, has gone to Germany to seek justice against Strippel by urging that he be brought to trial. This group, under the leadership of Henri Morgenstern, has participated in the annual services at the school building, demonstrated in the streets of Hamburg, and even sought out Strippel at his home in Frankfurt. Yet while they have through their activities brought their case forcefully before the conscience of the West German citizenry, they have still to convince German prosecutors to reopen a legal case against the former SS Kommandant. And until Arnold Strippel is brought to trial, Morgenstern says, the various commemorative tributes to the dead children will remain incomplete gestures.

In the meantime, though, there is Schwarberg's book. This English translation incorporates some new material supplied by the author that was not available to him at the time of the German publication and also includes some photographs that did not previously appear. Otherwise, apart from eliminating a very few passages written specifically with a German audience in mind, we have sought to translate Mr. Schwarberg's book in a way that would be faithful to the original and readily accessible to an American readership. In virtually all cases we have retained the author's use of SS ranks in the

German and have appended a glossary of equivalent U.S. Army ranks to help the reader get some approximate sense of the Nazi hierarchy. The glossary also lists a few other terms used to designate functionaries in the concentration camps.

We wish to thank Dr. Mark Wisen and Professor Craig Bradley, of Bloomington, Indiana, for their assistance in helping us with some of the more technical medical and legal language, and Weli Frishman, of Jerusalem, for his generous and pointed criticisms during the first reading of the book. Serge and Beate Klarsfeld, of Paris, proved helpful in supplying background information on Arnold Strippel and in informing us about the activities of "Les Fils et Filles de Déportés Juifs de France." The Klarsfelds also introduced us to Henri Morgenstern, who described the most recent efforts of his group in seeking to bring Strippel to trial. Tamar Laakmann, of Jerusalem, helped us obtain information about the museum and memorial rooms at the Bullenhuser Damm School, and Heinz-Günter Tessmer, the school principal, kindly answered our questions concerning recent commemorative arrangements. Finally, we wish to thank Patsy Ek for her speedy and accurate typing.

The translation and publication of this book were arranged by ZACHOR, the Holocaust Resource Center of the National Jewish Resource Center.

Alvin H. Rosenfeld
Erna B. Rosenfeld

As this book goes to press, the *New York Times* (December 13, 1983) has reported that on December 12 the Hamburg public prosecutor filed murder charges against Arnold Strippel for killing twenty Jewish children and twenty-two inmates of Neuengamme concentration camp in April 1945. The charges accused Strippel of hanging the children and killing other inmates to eliminate witnesses to medical experiments performed on the children. The charges came after a three-year investigation in France, Poland, Israel, and Czechoslovakia and included records from the British military government in 1945.

The Murders at Bullenhuser Damm

One

It was the week of the liberation of Paris. From the south the first troops of General Leclerc were bringing freedom to the capital of France. In the north, as the German troops were retreating, a final crime was committed.

On August 17, 1944, at 4:00 p.m., a transport of Jews left the train station of the Paris suburb of Bobigny on train number 1697. There were six cars, three holding antiaircraft guns, three carrying people. In the first car sat the staff of the secret police and its head, Alois Brunner, Hauptsturmführer of the SS. He was the head of the Sonderkommando in charge of deporting Jews in France. In the second car were members of the "Green Police," German police officials in green uniforms who operated in France.

The last car was a cattle car. Fifty-two Jews squatted inside, among them the seven members of the Kohn family. Alois Brunner knew them. Armand Kohn was a relative of the banker Rothschild and the director of the Baron de Rothschild Hospital in Paris, the largest Jewish hospital in France. During the German occupation Armand Kohn hid many Jews there who were allegedly seriously ill. Brunner had come to the clinic frequently. Now, he accused Armand Kohn of sabotage.

Nevertheless, Director Kohn felt that his personal dealings with Brunner would provide him with a certain amount of security, and he counted on Brunner to save his family from deportation.

But early in the morning of July 28, 1944, Brunner rang the doorbell at the Kohn house. Behind him stood the two SS men Samson and Reich. Brunner was polite: "Please pack your things. You are being deported. You have one hour." A Paris transit bus was waiting outside. It took the Kohns to the Jewish camp at Drancy.

On their arrival, all trace of politeness disappeared. Like all the other Jews, the Kohns were treated like prisoners condemned to

1

death. On August 17, 1944, they were taken from the camp to the train station.

Armand Kohn did not realize that deportation meant death. He knew about deportations. And he had heard the name Auschwitz. But despite everything he had heard, he believed that the Jews were only going to be interned until the end of the war. For that reason, he wanted to keep his family together. When his eighteen-year-old son, Philippe, wanted to escape from the train, Armand told his family that only by remaining together would they be protected. The son did not obey his father, nor did Philippe's sister Rose-Marie. The train had been moving for three days. On August 21, 1944, at 2:00 a.m., they broke the bars of the freight car's narrow windows and jumped. Rose-Marie went first—she injured herself on the railroad ties. Some sixty yards further on Philippe fell onto the tracks. Unhurt, he ran to his sister. Others followed them, among them the writer Jacques Lazarus and Rabbi Sami Kapelowitsch, who was later to become the Israeli ambassador to Paris, Jean ("Jeannot") Friedmann, and Henri ("Balou") Pohoryles. Thirty were able to flee, twelve remained. Among the latter, Armand Kohn and his wife, their nineteen-year-old daughter, Antoinette, and their twelve-year-old son, Georges André, born April 23, 1932. Those who escaped hid in a shallow pond so that the dogs of the SS would not find them. Later they were hidden by the stationmaster, who concealed them in the cellar of the Saint Quentin station until the liberation, on September 2, 1944.

As the train continued its journey, Armand Kohn dropped a note addressed to his secretary through a crack in the floor of the freight car:

> We are being deported and, without a doubt, are being sent to Germany. We trust in God. Try to do something for us through the International Red Cross! Try to meet with Pierre Taittinger, President of the Municipal Council of Paris. Au Revoir. Think of us. Tell all our friends and everyone at work.

The note was found near Villers-Cotterets, in the district of Aisne, and sent anonymously to Paris.

But this hope of being rescued was as great an illusion as Armand's belief that in staying together they would all be safe. On August 25, 1944, the train arrived at Buchenwald concentration camp, near Weimar. There the family was torn apart. The father stayed in Buchenwald; the grandmother and Georges were sent to Auschwitz; the mother and Antoinette, to Bergen-Belsen.

On the ramp at Auschwitz-Birkenau stood an SS doctor who pointed to the two Kohns and ordered them to go to the left. To the right were the gas chambers; to the left, the barracks. It was unusual for women and children to be sent to the barracks and not immediately to the gas chambers. As a rule, only men and strong boys were sent to the left—to work for six months until their death.

But Georges André Kohn was not put in the same barracks as his grandmother. Something special had been planned for him. For him and for nineteen other children.

What was intended for the children had been discussed three months earlier at the casino at Hohenlychen. This was a health spa run by the Red Cross in the Uckermark, about seventy miles north of Berlin, between Templin and Neustrelitz. At this old sanatorium situated on the beautiful Greater Lychensee, the SS leaders of nearby Ravensbrück concentration camp would rest from their work. It was here also that top SS officers met with politicians from Berlin, for Hohenlychen was a quiet place, safe from bombing attacks. Rudolf Hess, Hitler's deputy, came here often, as did the Nazi architect Albert Speer; the Minister of Sport for the Reich, Hans von Tschammer und Osten; the Propaganda Minister, Josef Goebbels; and Oswald Pohl, Obergruppenführer and General of the Waffen-SS. And, above all, Heinrich Himmler, Reichsführer of the SS, or RFSS, as he wanted to be called. Hitler himself had been here a few times. The SS had taken over the sanatorium in 1942.

One evening in the spring of 1944, the Reich's Minister of Health, Dr. Leonardo Conti, and Dr. Ernst Grawitz, Chief Physician of the SS and Police, gathered together with several colleagues. The Medical Director of Hohenlychen, Dr. Karl Gebhardt, gave the floor to his Assistant Director, Dr. Kurt Heissmeyer, for a short lecture.

Heissmeyer, thirty-eight at the time, had been a physician at Hohenlychen for the past ten years. To realize his aim of becoming a Professor of Medicine, he had to prepare and submit a scientific paper. He proposed to Dr. Conti an experiment relating to the fight against tuberculosis. The experiment was to be undertaken not with animals but with people. Heissmeyer had written in an earlier paper on "Self-Experimentation" that in the establishment of the philosophical theory of folk and race it is not feasible to deduce the origin of human tuberculosis from experiments on animals, for such a procedure suggests that the constitution of animals is the same as that of man. . . .

Now he wanted to test in practice the theory of two Austrian researchers on tuberculosis, A. and H. Kutschera-Aichbergen, a theory about "combatting severe tuberculosis of the lungs by artificially inducing tuberculosis of the skin."

In a number of publications between 1929 and 1939, these Austrians, father and son, had supported the view that the "immunity of a patient ill with active tuberculosis of the lungs" could be improved by "implanting" an additional tubercular node. Thus, one could hasten the healing process in the lungs and at least slow down the course of the illness if dead tubercle bacilli, or "tuberculin," were rubbed into scratches made in the skin.

However, eminent researchers in this area all over the world were by then already in agreement that the Kutschera-Aichbergen thesis was wrong. Yet Heissmeyer was ignorant of this, and the physicians to whom he delivered his lecture knew nothing of such research. In general, Heissmeyer's knowledge was very limited. He was a general practitioner and had never conducted any research. He regarded the Nazi teachings on race as a science.

In 1943 he had submitted a paper entitled "Principles of Present and Future Problems of TB Sanatoriums," in which he explained that "racially inferior" patients had lower resistance to illnesses such as tuberculosis than did racially superior ones. For this reason, he believed, doctors had to base their decisions about which patients to treat in a hospital on two things—"on the one hand, the importance of race, and on the other, the condition of the organ itself." By the "condition of the organ" Heissmeyer meant what physicians the world over mean by "diagnosis." But to him, considerations of race came first.

Following Heissmeyer's lecture, Professor Gebhardt asked Dr. Conti whether Heissmeyer could try his experiments on prisoners in Ravensbrück concentration camp, most of whom were women. Professor Gebhardt himself had had some experience with human experiments. He had artificially produced gas gangrene wounds in the women and practiced bone transplants on them. Conti gave his permission, as did Grawitz. Heissmeyer was told he should get Himmler's permission to undertake these experiments. The two doctors would support this request.

Hitler had already decided in 1942 that "as a matter of principle, if it is in the interest of the state, human experiments were to be permitted," and prisoners could be used for that purpose. For it was wrong that "someone in a concentration camp or prison be totally untouched by the war, while German soldiers had to suffer the unbearable, and while the homeland, together with women and children, was being destroyed by fire bombs."[1] Himmler, however, had given orders that human experiments were to be carried out only with his permission.

As a defendant at the doctors' trial in Nuremberg, Professor Gebhardt made the following statement:

> Himmler's whole aspiration was to develop a science that belonged uniquely to the SS. . . . Those individuals who were graduates of universities or those trained as health officers resisted, of course, everything new instituted by the Third Reich but would have been prepared perhaps to discuss changing the tone or the content of what already existed. But there was a certain group of people in the Third Reich—people like Himmler and Hess—who believed that nothing new or vibrant could come out of this tired bourgeois earth and that new ways would have to be charted, using young and still dormant talents. Himmler founded a group called the "Friends of Himmler," to which I never belonged. It was that dangerous mix of individualists and people from industry. And from this group Himmler obtained the money as well as the drive for the thousands of experiments he carried out in all areas.[2]

The year before the end of the war, however, Himmler had every reason to have human experiments be conducted only with his permission: the talkative Professor Gebhardt had been telling everyone that he was carrying out such experiments on women prisoners. In May 1943, he even gave a lecture on "Specific Experiments on the Effects of Sulfonamide" before two hundred consulting physicians of the Wehrmacht at the Berlin Military Academy of Medicine. That is how other countries learned that German doctors were treating prisoners as guinea pigs and killing them. The indignation that this aroused was embarrassing to Himmler, for at this time, and without Hitler's knowledge, he was holding talks with Count Folke Bernadotte of Sweden about the possibility of an armistice with the Western powers.

And so Heissmeyer had to win over Himmler if he was to carry out his human experiments on concentration camp inmates. To be sure, Heissmeyer was not considered scientifically qualified: a paper of his on the "Theory of Exhaustion" (to the effect that only "exhausted" and "inferior" organisms could be infected with tubercle bacilli) had been rejected by experts as inadequate.

But Heissmeyer had good connections. He was a friend of SS-General Oswald Pohl, who as head of the SS Economic and Administrative Office oversaw all concentration camps. And he also had an uncle who had contact with many important Nazi politicians: August Heissmeyer was a general of the Waffen-SS and Police, head of the Reich's Security Service, Inspector of "Napolas" (National Political Educational Institutes), and, above all, he was married to Gertrud Scholz-Klink, the head of the Women's League of the Reich.

There is no proof that this uncle spoke with Himmler about his nephew's intended plans for conducting human experiments, but it is improbable that such a conversation did not take place. At any rate, Himmler agreed, and Oswald Pohl relayed as much, in a second conversation at Hohenlychen, to his friend Dr. Kurt Heissmeyer. However, Pohl requested that the experiments not take place at Ravensbrück, where Gebhardt had already aroused so much undesirable attention, but rather at a more discreet location. Pohl and Heissmeyer settled on Neuengamme concentration camp, near Hamburg.

In the last week of April, 1944, Kurt Heissmeyer went for the first time with Dr. Enno Lolling, Director of the Health Institute of the SS, to his new place of work. Heissmeyer wore a dark blue civilian suit, even though he was a ranking SS officer. The prisoners were to see him only as a doctor. Lagerkommandant Max Pauly introduced his staff to the two doctors from Hohenlychen; and, most important, Heissmeyer also met Dr. Alfred Trzebinski, Standortarzt, or Senior Physician, at Neuengamme, who would be supervising the experiments for him.

These gentlemen made the rounds of the crowded camp. Pauly, always proud of his technical organization, showed them Barracks 4a and the rear section of Sickbay 4, which had already been prepared for Heissmeyer's experiments. The area was especially marked off by a wooden fence. The windows were painted white. None of the prisoners was to see what was happening in this "Special Section Heissmeyer." All contact between the human guinea pigs and the other inmates of the camp was forbidden.

Heissmeyer returned to Hohenlychen well satisfied. The human experiments could begin.

But Georges André Kohn still had a reprieve at Birkenau. Heissmeyer planned to experiment first with adults and only later with children.

Upon arrival in Auschwitz, Georges Kohn was put in Barracks 11 of Block B I a in the Birkenau camp. How things were when one got there he was never able to report. But we have a description from a Polish girl his age, Gisa Landau, from Tarnow, who was liberated by the Red Army. She had arrived in Auschwitz on October 21, 1944, at the same time as Georges Kohn. This is what she reported:

> Cramped together and choking for air we rode in closed boxcars. We said good-bye to one another because we knew that the ovens and the gas chambers were waiting for us. Even though we often spoke about it, no one could really imagine what it would be like. When we got to Auschwitz at night we were herded off to Birkenau. In the distance we already noticed the sky as red as if it were on fire. Even though we had already gone through a lot, none of us could imagine that human beings should be burnt. There was no smoke coming out of the chimneys, just a rain of fire. People asked the guards what was burning, and they said that "after all, bread had to be baked day and night." But we knew that this could not be the case.
>
> At night we sat in a large room. It was so horrible that I cannot describe it. We cried, prayed, and sat there numb. Some of us were already totally indifferent. My mother pressed me close to her and whispered that I mustn't be afraid, for God would surely save us as He had until now. I didn't want to make her sad so I acted as if I was not afraid. In reality my whole body was shaking with fear. We didn't get anything to eat, nor did we feel any hunger. Why should we eat if we were going to have to die anyway? Then they made the selection. It was ghastly. We had to undress completely. Dr. Mengele[3] stood at the door and determined who should live and who should die. . . . We went into the bath, where our heads were shaved and where we had a number tattooed on us. I got number A 26 098. Getting a num-

ber at all was considered good—almost as good as being saved. Unfortunately, children were selected time and again and sent to the ovens.

Georges Kohn did not have a number tattooed on him. They saved themselves the effort because he was to go into the "Special Section Heissmeyer"; he was singled out by the same Dr. Josef Mengele, from Günzberg, who had also "selected" Gisa Landau.

In Barracks 11 other children had already been assembled, both boys and girls, the youngest five years old, the oldest ones as old as Georges. Almost all spoke Polish. But Georges did find another child from Paris—a girl named Jacqueline Morgenstern, who was also twelve years old.

Jacqueline's father and uncle had owned a beauty shop near the Place de la République. Originally, they had come from Czernowitz, in the Romanian Bukovina, leaving their home for France as anti-Semitism was becoming more and more oppressive. The brothers learned French, but at home they spoke German, the language spoken for many generations in the Bukovina. When the Germans came to Paris in 1940 the brothers Morgenstern had to hand over their shop to a non-Jewish Frenchman. One brother, Leopold, was arrested in Paris by the French police, while his pregnant wife, Dorothéa, succeeded in escaping with their two children. The other brother, Karl Morgenstern, fled with his wife, Suzanne, and his daughter, Jacqueline, to Marseille, a part of France not yet occupied by the Germans. They had forged papers. For a time they hid in a back room at the home of an aunt. But someone denounced them one day to the Gestapo. The Morgensterns were arrested and taken from the south of France to the large Jewish collection camp at Drancy.

On June 20, 1944, they were transported by train to Auschwitz; it was Convoy No. 74, with 565 men, 632 women, and 191 children. On arrival, 188 men were immediately taken off the ramp and sent to the right, into the gas chambers. Jacqueline and her parents were spared for the time being. But they were separated. Her father was put in the men's camp, Jacqueline and her mother in the women's camp. Suzanne Morgenstern, who had worked as a secretary in Paris, became weaker and weaker, since she gave most of her rations to young Jacqueline. Finally she contracted dysentery and soon thereafter was also sent to the gas chambers. Karl Morgenstern must have learned of the killing of his wife before he died. He remained in Auschwitz until it was dissolved, but in January 1945, before the Red Army liberated the camp he was taken with the last transport to Dachau—in an open freight car, without any provisions. When he arrived there he was deathly ill, emaciated, and had gone mad. He was still alive, however, when the Americans came, but only for a few days. On May 23, 1945, he died in Feldafing Hospital.

After the murder of her mother, Jacqueline was kept in Children's Barracks No. 11. There she found Georges Kohn; they would be friends for the rest of their short lives.

It was remarkable that these twenty children were allowed to live. Their barracks were heated, their meals were almost sufficient. The Polish nurses who lived with them sang them songs, comforted them, and taught them games. They took them in their arms when the children cried with longing for their parents, who were no longer alive. And they tried to distract them from the horrible smell spread by the heavy dark clouds coming from the crematorium. It smelled "like burning flesh, as if a goose were getting scorched in an oven, only much stronger." This is how it was described by Krystyna Zywulska, who was liberated from Birkenau by the Red Army in January 1945.[4]

An SS-Unterscharführer, Oswald Kaduk, who was Rapportführer in Auschwitz, also remembered the smell. Sentenced for life to Schwalmstadt prison, he commented:

> My son came to visit me once on a Sunday. He was about eight or ten years old. . . . And he asked me, "Daddy, why does it smell so bad here?" What could I tell the boy? . . . I told him it was the Wistula River, or the water, or this or that, but he did know and my wife did too.[5]

Jacqueline Morgenstern and Georges André Kohn could communicate with the other children only with difficulty, even though they were the same age. Among their companions were a Polish girl, Lelka Birnbaum, and a Yugoslav boy named Junglieb, both twelve, and ten-year-old Marek Steinbaum, from Poland.

They could more easily understand the Dutch spoken by the two Hornemann brothers—twelve-year-old Eduard (called Edo) and eight-year-old Alexander (nicknamed Lexje). Both were emaciated. They had just seen their mother, Elisabeth Hornemann, die of typhoid fever at the end of September 1944, in Birkenau. She was thirty-seven. And they had not seen their father for a long time, even though he was also at Birkenau, in the men's camp.

Gradually the boys regained their strength, due to the better care given the "Heissmeyer children." After all, healthy children were needed for the experiments. Lexje even regained the happy naïveté of the little clown he had been. Children who had gone to school with him in Eindhoven before his deportation still remember anecdotes about him today. For example, he once went up to his math teacher, shook hands, and wished her a good day—all of which was against school regulations. They also recall that when he was given the Jewish star on his sixth birthday, on May 31, 1942, he was very proud to wear it on his jacket and showed it off as if it were a present. This made a deep impression on his Dutch classmates. They knew more about this star than the happy, naïve Lexje Hornemann.

His parents also did not consider the danger seriously enough at that time. His father, Philip Carel ("Flip") Hornemann, was a buyer for Philips in Eindhoven. After Holland was occupied by the German Wehrmacht and the Jewish deportations began, this corporation set up a special section for Jewish employees called SOBU (Special Development Bureau). They produced measuring instruments essential to the German occupation army for the war effort. At the end of 1941, Flip Hornemann was put in SOBU with about a hundred other Philips employees. Because they thought they were protected by the power of a large corporation, the Jews felt a greater sense of security from being seized by German patrols.

At this time the management did indeed do much to give its employees the feeling of being part of a large family. When the Germans arrested the owner of the firm, Frits Philips, Flip Hornemann told his children about it with such concern that six-year-old Alexander was moved to pray for his father's employer every night. The security that the SOBU workers felt was deceptive, however, and came to an end on August 18, 1943, when German troops surrounded SOBU in Eindhoven and arrested all the Jews. Immediately the news spread throughout the city. Elisabeth Hornemann ran to the factory and just managed to see her husband being put in an open truck. She was able to embrace him, and he whispered, "Go into hiding!" Then the Germans drove them off to the Dutch concentration camp Vught near s'Hertogenbosch.

This camp established its own Philips operation with over 3,000 prisoners. The Jews from SOBU were once again to turn out measuring instruments. The Philips workers received somewhat better food—the "Philips stew"—than the other camp inmates. They were also better protected from the cruelty of the SS and its brutal Schutzhaftlagerführer, Arnold Strippel. And they were given the special privilege of living together with their wives and children, if the latter joined them.

Two days after the SOBU Jews were interned, the women and children who wanted to be with their husbands were told to get ready. Elisabeth Hornemann thought that less harm would come to them under the protection of the Philips company than if she continued to live with her two boys outside the concentration camp. But then she had a visit from a friend of the family, old Pastor Vonk from the village of Aarle-Rixtel, near Eindhoven. He implored her to hide in the pigsty on his farm, like her sister Ans. While he was trying to persuade her, two men from Philips arrived and told her she simply had to go with them to the camp; otherwise, the firm could not guarantee her safety. This discussion of life or death went on for two hours. Neighbors later recalled how Elisabeth Hornemann ran back and forth crying, not knowing whether to go or to stay.

Finally she wrote a note to her sister in hiding and gave it to Pastor Vonk. It read:

> Dear ones, it is 11 a.m. Friday morning. The bus will come any moment now. I can't make up my mind. The Philips people have tried to persuade me; they're still so optimistic. I've decided to go with them, although I don't share their hope. They told me I was the only one who didn't want to go along. They did everything to dissuade me from my original decision. It was unbelievable how our friend Vonk talked with them. I was at wit's end. Now I'll try to be strong and go. Flip is going to be surprised to see me. I am leaving—what do you say to that? But I'll be back.

When the bus from Philips came and stopped in front of the Hornemann house on Gagelstraat 49, Mrs. Hornemann got her boys into their coats, and they all boarded the bus.

Her husband was horrified when he saw them get off the bus. "Why did you come? You should have stayed away!" He suspected the worst. The SOBU Jews remained in the Vught camp only until

June 3, 1944, then they too had to board the deportation train. On
the day they stood on the ramps in Birkenau—June 9, 1944—the
Allies had landed on the coast of Normandy.

The men were separated from the women. The children remained with their mothers. The men were sent to the work barracks,
the women and children to the showers. Some of them had heard of
the gas chambers, and now they waited naked for their death. But the
shower heads produced no Cyclon-B, just water. Real warm water. It
was incredible that there were showers in Birkenau that were nothing
but showers. After they had their hair cut off they were returned to
the barracks. Three months later Elisabeth Hornemann became ill
with typhoid fever. Her two children stood outside the infirmary
every day.

A fellow Dutch inmate in the camp, Lena Goslinski-Frank, reported after she was freed that she had met Edo and Lexje outside the
sickbay:

> Both were sick, and Lexje was so thin that I didn't recognize him
> at first. The boys told me that their mother was in the hospital.
> Later I didn't hear anything more from them. Judging from the
> conditions I found them in at the time, I assume they both died
> soon after our meeting.

A few days after their mother's death, both boys were asked to
step forward at the morning roll call in front of their barracks and
were taken away. "That was a striking moment," Hetty Lissauer, who
had come to the camp as a nine-year-old, said, describing the scene.
"That had never happened before, and we never found out what it
was all about."

The Hornemann children had been chosen for Dr. Heissmeyer's
experiments. From that moment on, none of the Dutch inmates ever
saw the two boys or their father again. On January 17, 1945, as
Auschwitz and Birkenau were being evacuated, and before the Red
Army liberated the camps, Philip Carel Hornemann died. He was
riding in an open freight car, wearing only thin prison garb, in zero
degree weather.

Even though none of the twenty children has left us a description
of life in Birkenau, we know it fairly well. For near Barracks 11 there
was another children's barracks where SS-Doctor Josef Mengele kept
a group of Jewish twins and used them in experiments. He wanted to
determine through different tests what characteristics twins held in

common. Like his SS colleague, Heissmeyer, he hoped, through establishing his own "Theory of Twins," to become a Professor of Medicine.

A Polish nurse, Elzbieta Piekut-Warszawska, who survived Birkenau together with about one hundred of the "Mengele children," described what went on in Mengele's barracks:

> There was a brick oven running the length of a wooden building. Inside the room were wooden bunks. The children were of Jewish origin and came from different countries—France, Holland, Belgium, Hungary, and Germany. On arrival they were still healthy and pretty, only somewhat frightened and tearful. Depending on their age, they slept in bunks by two's or four's, on straw mats but without sheets or pillows. Each bunk had two blankets. Their food consisted of black campbread, margarine (on Sunday white bread with jam), a black coffee substitute, milk soup, noodles, cheese. . . . The three of us had to wash the children daily in small basins with very little water. The older children helped us.[6]

TWO

Georges Kohn and Jacqueline Morgenstern were fortunate to come into contact with other deportees from France who helped them and cheered them up. Louis Micard, a prisoner from Rouen, writing after the war to Georges's brother Philippe, who had survived, recalls:

> We all received Georges with love. We all tried to make him forget where he was and to ease the anxiety he felt at being separated from his mother. . . . Weeks passed. A selection of children took place. Georges looked very weak, and we feared that he would be selected. Friends, who were French doctors in the sickbay where this selection was taking place, succeeded in getting him through by ingenious means.
>
> Bad days were upon us. Winter, snow, wind, and cold were our enemies. But Georges was all right. He had warm clothing and solid shoes—a rarity—to keep his feet dry. He worked at loading the "dumpcarts" with refuse, or firewood, or sometimes coal. The Kapo was German; he screamed a lot but was not too mean, and he didn't hit. . . . I then lost track of young Georges. He was a very nice boy, and we all thought of him as our little brother.

Dr. Albert Vogel, a French physician from Neuilly-sur-Seine, wrote after the war:

> I worked as a doctor in a block, just like such other colleagues as Dr. August and Dr. Desiré Hafner. We tried to help the little Kohn boy both physically and by lifting his morale. During our stay in Birkenau he was doing quite well, and he was relatively happy in our company. He visited me often in my block, and I was thus able to learn of the odyssey of the unfortunate Kohn family.

14

Like the "Mengele children," those in Barracks 11 also had to go to the infirmary for medical examinations. "This was an ordeal for the children," Elzbieta Piekut-Warszawska writes.

> Frightened, tired, hungry, and numb with cold they had to get up at six in the morning and walk almost a mile from their block to the infirmary. . . . It was already quite cool—the end of September, the beginning of October—and the examination room was not heated. The children who were being examined had to line up naked in front of the X-ray screen, for anywhere from five to fifteen minutes because the doctors would discuss each X-ray as it was being viewed through the fluoroscope. . . . When they returned to their block, the children became feverish, contracted angina, a heavy cough, sinus inflammations, and often pneumonia.[1]

A throat culture report from one of these examinations exists, despite the destruction of virtually all written evidence when the camp was evacuated. This card is the only document that remains today in the Auschwitz Museum charting the suffering of the imprisoned Heissmeyer children. It shows that on May 14, 1944, a throat culture was taken of Sergio de Simone, an Italian child born November 29, 1937, Auschwitz number 179614. He and his parents, Eduardo and Gisela de Simone, née Perlow, had come to Auschwitz as part of a transport that had been dispatched from a collection center for Italian Jews in Trieste.

Children too understand death when they see pillars of fire rising up daily from the chimneys of the crematoria. Dr. Otto Wolken, a Viennese pediatrician, was one of the prison doctors at that time. After the war he wrote "When I Think about the Children,"[2] in which he tells of a nine-year-old boy from Poland who told the doctor just before he was sent to the gas chamber:

> My shoes are still very good. Maybe you can find someone who wants to exchange them with me for a bread ration. I won't need them anymore. I'm sure I won't. And I would really like to eat my fill once more before I die.

For the children death was an everyday affair. It took place not only in the gas chambers, it appeared in many different shapes as well. One such ghastly form was the children's disease called noma (gangrenous stomatitis), which ravaged the faces of the starving children with a cancerlike growth. Even the SS people were afraid of it. Lagerkommandant Rudolf Höss describes how he took Reichsführer-SS Heinrich Himmler on a tour of the camp in 1942 and showed him these dying children:

> We had a visit by the RFSS in July 1942. I showed him the gypsy camp. He inspected everything very carefully; he saw the cramped living conditions, the lack of hygiene, the crowded infirmaries, the patients with infectious diseases, the children's disease noma, which made me shudder every time. It reminded me of the lepers whom I had once seen in Palestine—those emaciated children with gaping holes in their cheeks that one could see through, the slow rotting away of living flesh.[3]

But children take into their lives even the death that surrounds them. They use it in their games. Hanna Hofmann-Fischel reported:

> They played *"Lagerältester"* and *"Blockältester,"* "Roll Call," shouting "Caps off!" They took on the roles of the sick who fainted during roll call and were beaten for it; or they played "Doctor"—a doctor who would take away food rations from the sick and refuse them all help if they had nothing to bribe him with. Once they even played "Gas Chamber." They made a hole in the ground and threw in stones one after the other. Those were supposed to be people put in the crematoria, and they imitated their screams. They wanted me to show them how to set up the chimney.[4]

Some of the bigger boys also played games of daring. They approached the electric fence, some even touching it lightning-quick with the tips of their fingers. They were lucky—for the most part the current was shut off during the day.

Georges Kohn may well have had the chance to see the gas chambers during the time he was working with the dumpcarts. Jehuda Bacon, from Mährisch-Ostrau, one of the other boys who did this heavy work as part of the dumpcart crew, describes the scene. He was three years older than Georges.

> I became part of the so-called dumpcart kommando. It consisted of a wagon pulled by twenty youngsters instead of by horses. That's how I got around the whole camp. I knew exactly what was going on in Auschwitz. We even got into the women's

camp and frequently into the crematorium. It was our job to distribute blankets and laundry; but above all we had to bring some of the wood that was near the gas chamber—it was needed for the cremations—over to the camp for use there. I remember the Kapo once telling us in the winter: "Boys, you've finished loading up. If you want to get a little warm, go in the gas chamber. There's no one in there right now."

And so it happened that we were able to get a look at the gas chambers, the ovens, the whole installation—above all, underground Crematorium 2. We were young then and interested in everything. I once said to one of the Sonderkommandos: "Come on, tell me everything; maybe I'll get out, and then I'll write about you."

They just laughed and said that no one got out of there alive. But they told me a lot all the same. Underground Crematoria 1 and 2 were very modern structures. First you had to go to a room to get undressed—that's what the member of the Sonderkommando told me. (Of course, I myself was never in there when a transport arrived. We sometimes stood outside and were told not to go in because there were people in there.) The people had to get undressed. There were hooks marked with numbers on the walls. The SS used to tell the people: "Fold your clothes neatly and remember your number so that you can get your things back on the other side, after the disinfection." Many asked for coffee, for they were so thirsty after their long trip. The SS man would only hurry them along saying, "Be quick about it or your coffee will get cold. Your coffee is waiting for you back in the camp."

When the people were undressed they were herded into the gas chambers. At first glance one would think the gas chamber was a real shower. But I was very curious and looked at it more closely. And so I discovered that the holes on what would be the shower head were only faked. Behind them there were openings for ventilators. The lamps on the ceiling were covered with wire mesh. Two cagelike structures running from the middle of the ceiling down to the floor were also covered with similar wire mesh, sixteen inches square.

When everything was ready an SS man poured Cyclon-B into these cages from an opening in the ceiling of the gas chamber. After a time, when everyone was dead, an automatic ventilation system went on. And later the Sonderkommandos came, took out the dead, and threw them onto an open lift that brought them up to the first floor. From there the corpses were taken in trolleys to the ovens, where they were burned. Prior to this a special kommando would also knock out the victims' gold teeth. Sometimes their hair would be shaved off as well, if this had not already been done earlier.[5]

Yet this fear of death that everyone in Birkenau lived with would alternate time and again with feelings of hope. Even though there were no newspapers or radios, even the children knew that the liberators were drawing nearer. In July 1944, the Soviet soldiers had liberated Majdanek concentration camp near Lublin, 180 miles from Auschwitz and Birkenau. By the end of October 1944, the Red Army was outside Cracow, only 35 miles to the east.

All at once the gasings stopped. The crematoria were torn down. A foreman named Koch, employed by J. A. Topf and Sons[6] Furnace Manufacturing Company of Erfurt, was in charge of the dismantling and had the steel parts of the structures loaded onto a freight train. The most modern machine in the world for cremating corpses—with a capacity of burning up to 7,000 human beings per day—was to be reassembled in another German concentration camp, possibly Gross-Rosen.

Suddenly an explosion shook the camp at Birkenau. Some of the inmates thought it was the Americans beginning the long-awaited attack on the death factory. But it was the SS instead, blowing up the walls of the gas chambers. The end of Birkenau and Auschwitz was near—an end that had to bring the prisoners either death or freedom.[7] Then the order came from Berlin: Heissmeyer needed the children in Neuengamme now.

In early June, 1944, Dr. Heissmeyer had begun his experiments in Neuengamme concentration camp—at first with adults and in absolute secrecy. No one was permitted to enter the "Heissmeyer Barracks" except the experimental subjects, a German orderly, Herbert Kirst, and two French inmate doctors, Professor Florence and Professor Quenouille. No one was permitted to discuss the experiments, on pain of death. But they were discussed all the same.

Every Wednesday Heissmeyer came from Hohenlychen to Neuengamme, 165 miles away. He always wore a dark blue civilian suit. The first time he came he brought with him a glass bottle containing a strain of live, virulent, and therefore infectious tubercle bacilli. He had obtained them from the laboratory of Professor Meinicke, a bacteriologist from Berlin. The latter knew nothing about Heissmeyer's experiments. But the request for this bacteria had come from the SS, and Dr. Meinicke therefore warned Heissmeyer about testing them on people. Human testing is admissable at most only with dead tubercle bacilli. Heissmeyer assured him he was not planning any human testing.

Heissmeyer later testified before the interrogation officers:

> When I received the serum, I was cautioned by Meinicke to be absolutely sure to test it on animals first in order to determine its effects. This, in fact, is what I did. However, during the whole course of the testing, I injected only twelve animals in all with the serum, even though I knew that this number was totally insufficient. Besides, the animal testing ran parallel to the testing of the inmates. Meinicke had advised me to observe the guinea pigs that I would inject for at least three to four months, because only then could the effect of the serum be determined with any measure of certainty.
>
> But I did not do this, because I wanted to have the results of the use of serum on humans in as short a time as possible. There-fore, soon after receiving the serum, I injected a number of adult prisoners at Neuengamme (I no longer remember how many); in other words, I did not await the results of the animal testing. Being a doctor, I knew, of course, that I was not allowed to do this, for it was after all a virulent serum that I was injecting. Thus I was knowingly exposing human subjects to the danger of con-tracting TB and at the same time endangering the lives of the prisoners and later the lives of the children. In this connection it can be said that in the case of tuberculosis every prognosis is unpredictable. I also took into account that if things turned out badly the human subjects would die as a result of being injected with the TB serum. This would be the case, since at that time there were still no medicines available of the kind whose applica-tion today enhances the prospects of recovery. But on the other hand, I mostly used prisoners for the experiments who were already very ill with TB. I knew that this testing would make them worse and that their chances of survival were extremely slim.[8]

The bottle containing the deadly bacilli strain was kept in Heissmeyer's "lab" in Barracks 4; there the solutions for the injections were prepared from the strain. Heissmeyer showed Kirst how to do this: according to his discretion Kirst was to take some of the bacteria culture with an inoculating loop and grind it together with a saline solution in a porcelain mortar. Heissmeyer did not know that this was life-threatening work, to be done only while wearing protective masks. "He was also ignorant of the proper ways of handling bacteria," Professor Otto Prokop, Director of the Institute for Forensic Medicine at Humboldt University in East Berlin, testified later.

> The cultures that were used were lying around in the laboratory. Thus it was possible for one of the French doctors to inactivate the cultures by boiling so as to make them harmless. . . . Nor did Heissmeyer determine the dose of these bacterial inoculations.[9]

Heissmeyer had the solution brought to him in the X-ray room of Sickbay Barracks 1, where Kirst had prepared a prisoner for the experiment. The inmate had to sit on a stool, and Heissmeyer inserted a rubber tube down the prisoner's trachea into his lungs. This was very painful and caused a strong fit of coughing. At times Heissmeyer damaged the windpipe and caused bleeding. Many prisoners would scream.

Then the person had to step behind the X-ray screen. Heissmeyer checked the position of the probe, took the first X-ray picture, and then injected the tubercle solution into the lobes of the lungs. These prisoners were mostly very emaciated young men, Russians and Poles, between twenty and thirty years old. A few weighed just seventy-five to a hundred pounds. As long as they were in the "Special Section Heissmeyer," however, they were given better food—white bread, for example. This was generally known in the camp, and there were inmates who even volunteered for Heissmeyer's section. Heissmeyer said later:

> I know nothing about people reporting voluntarily, but I do remember that some prisoners did not want to leave my barracks because their diet was relatively good compared to conditions in the rest of the camp—all in the interest of the experiments.[10]

The SS doctor could select anyone he wanted for his experiments, for not only Lagerkommandant Pauly but all the other SS personnel in the camp knew of Heissmeyer's good connections with Berlin and with the top echelon of the SS. It was never learned how many adults fell into Heissmeyer's hands, but there must have been over a hundred. The medical records of thirty-two experimental subjects have been preserved.

In his experiments, Heissmeyer injected tubercle suspensions not only into the lungs but also under the skin. Some prisoners had tubercular sputum rubbed into scratches made in the skin.

At first Heissmeyer experimented on a group of patients who suffered from severe bilateral tuberculosis of the lungs, then with a group that had tuberculosis in only one lobe. The third group was free of TB of the lungs but suffered the disease in other organs. And finally Heissmeyer gathered together at random a number of healthy prisoners, free of TB, to serve as the "control group." These at least knew that they were made ill here. The others might have been led to believe that the doctor was trying to cure them. But the truth is, they all faced death.

At his hearings, Heissmeyer was later asked what he told his test subjects about the nature of the experiments. Heissmeyer:

> In answering this question I must admit that I did not tell them anything about the character and purpose of the experiments, nor the dangers connected with them. This was, in any case, not necessary, because as inmates of the concentration camp they had no rights whatsoever, and given the existing conditions in the camp, they were more or less forced to be at my disposal if I felt they were suitable for the experiments.[11]

Heissmeyer saw the results of his testing when the autopsies were performed. After observing for four weeks how the patients first developed a high fever and how the tubercular nodes spread in the lungs, he told his colleague Trzebinski that the experiments were completed. The following day—"Heissmeyer Day"—he found the freshly hanged corpses of his patients in the morgue, ready for section. The same thing also happened on November 8, 1944, with the following four inmates: Nedza, Wesselowsky, Wolniewicz, and Iwan Tschurkin, a locksmith from Kalinin who had just turned twenty-two a few days before.

Later, at his interrogation, Heissmeyer said that in the fall of 1944 he himself realized that the condition of the inmates used in these tests had worsened in all cases. He also realized about the same time that inoculations with live tubercle bacilli could not cure the TB but only make it worse.

At his interrogation, Heissmeyer added:

After determining in the fall of 1944 that my plan to heal TB
patients with the aforementioned serum had failed, and that the
condition of most of the inmates had worsened and not improved
(I no longer remember how many inmates were involved), I dis-
continued the experiments. I then ordered twenty children to be
brought in, on whom I used the same serum to see if they were
inherently immune to TB as well as to see if I could immunize
them against the disease.[12]

Although the continuation of the experiments had become senseless even for Heissmeyer, he went on with them all the same. He
wanted to complete his research, and one experimental group was
still lacking: the children.

Three

We have a protocol that describes the transport of the children from Auschwitz to Neuengamme. Dr. Pauline Trocki was born in Kishinev on December 28, 1905, moved to Belgium in 1923, and was active in the resistance there. As a result, she was arrested and taken to Auschwitz. After the war she emigrated to Israel and, until her death, lived in Givatayim. On December 30, 1956, she spoke the following for the record:[1]

One day I was summoned to the Lagerführer at noon and told I was to accompany a transport of children. Besides me, there were three nurses, one of them a laboratory technician from Hungary. The transport consisted of ten boys and ten girls between the ages of six and twelve. All were Jews, and they came from different countries; two were from Paris. I asked why the children were being transferred. They said these children had no parents. But I learned from the children themselves that many of their parents had been in the labor camp and had been sent off from there. An SS man accompanied the twenty children, one doctor, and three nurses to Neuengamme. A special railroad car was attached to a regular train, and from the outside everything seemed normal. During the trip we had to remove our Jewish stars so that we would not be conspicuous. To keep others from making contact with us it was said that this was a transport of typhoid patients.

The transport included a twelve-year-old boy, the son of Dr. Kohn, who, as I recall, was the director of the Rothschild Hospital in Paris. When the child saw Berlin from the train, he said: "If I knew somebody here I would escape." His father had been sent to Buchenwald with the last transport out of Paris.

We were given excellent food along the way, including

chocolate and milk. In two days we arrived at Neuengamme. It was night. I noticed someone cry when he saw the children. I spoke with a medical student from Belgium.[2] He said, "I'm afraid they intend to use the children in experiments. But there's a French doctor here, Dr. Florence. He will try to save them." This medical student worked in the pharmacy.

I never saw the children again.

On November 29, 1944, the transport arrived at Neuengamme, on a railroad spur that led directly into the camp. It was three days before the first Sunday of Advent.

Everything was in readiness for the children. Barracks 4a was heated; every child had his own bed in the double bunks—a luxury in the concentration camp. The four men who would be tending the children from this point on were put up in the hall. They were Dirk Deutekom and Anton Hölzel, two Dutch orderlies, and René Quenouille and Gabriel Florence, two French professors of medicine.

Neuengamme was essentially a camp for men. There was only one special barracks for women. The woman doctor and the three Polish nurses were placed in the back rooms of this special barracks.

Ruth Schemmel, from Hamburg, a housewife who was one of the prisoners in this barracks at the time, reports:

Two of the women were very thin; they were between forty-five and fifty-five years old. One was a physician, the other a pharmacologist. The two younger ones were Poles, between twenty and thirty years old, and they seemed to be in better physical shape. Their hair was short—as if it had been shaved off at one time and now had grown back. They said they had accompanied the children here from Auschwitz and thought they would be allowed to stay with them. They had only small bags with them containing toothbrushes and washcloths; otherwise, they had nothing. The first Sunday of Advent we celebrated together; we had a few evergreen branches for the occasion. One evening Rapportführer Wilhelm Dreimann came and said to me, "As of tomorrow the new arrivals won't be getting any more food. They're going to be moved." On Tuesday he came for them. The women took their bags, and I said good-bye to them. Then they went off in the direction of the prison barracks.

The doctor was sent to Bendorf concentration camp, near Magdeburg. It is not known what happened to the nurses.

Later, on March 27, 1946, Michel Müller, a former inmate, described before the British Military Tribunal the execution in 1944 of four Polish women in Neuengamme. It is not certain that the three nurses were among them, but they could well have been.

> Müller: "In 1944 four Polish women were hanged in the prison barracks. These women resisted with all their might, because they were to undress completely. They screamed terribly. The prisoners at the building site heard them but did not know what was going on."
> Prosecutor: "We want to know what Pauly had to do with this."

SS-Obersturmbannführer Max Pauly, thirty-seven years old, father of five children, was Kommandant of the Neuengamme concentration camp.

> Müller: "Kommandant Pauly was present at every execution in the prison barracks. One of the four women was pregnant. At Pauly's request her body was dissected because he wanted to see one time how that event was taking place in a woman's body. Dr. Adolf did all the explaining."
> Prosecutor: "You said this was in 1944. Where were you during this time?"
> Müller: "I had to take down the body."
> Prosecutor: "How do you know about the autopsy?"
> Müller: "The next morning I was at the area bath, and there I saw a prison-hand sew the body up again from top to bottom. There were two women in every coffin. Two prison orderlies told me that Pauly had said he wanted to know what pregnancy in a woman looked like. Dr. Adolf explained everything to him."[3]

Kommandant Pauly denied at the trial that he had been present at the dissection. He maintained that he reprimanded the camp physician, Dr. Adolf, for doing a section on a pregnant woman.

It can no longer be determined on which day Heissmeyer inoculated the children for the first time with the tubercle bacilli, nor how many of them were subjected to that painful inoculation with the lung probe; in any case, not all of them were.

Later, when some of the X-ray photos were found, Professor Schubert, radiologist of the Charité in Berlin, ascertained that Jacqueline Morgenstern, the Polish girl Lelka Birnbaum, and the seven-year-old Italian boy Sergio de Simone all had "infiltrative changes" in the lobes of the lungs—typical of Heissmeyer's "innoculations."

All the children had incisions made in their skin into which the tubercle cultures were rubbed, and all of the children contracted a fever within two or three days.

Georges André Kohn was especially weakened, and from this time on he was no longer able to get up, even though everyone tried very hard to look after him. Because they shared the same language, the two French professors were often with the two French children, sitting at their bedside as Jacqueline and Georges told them their sad stories of how they got to the camp, while the two doctors told them theirs in turn.

Professor René Quenouille was then sixty. Until March 3, 1943, he had practiced radiology in Villeneuve-Saint-Georges, near Paris. On that day he was arrested by the French police because he had tried to hide British paratroopers. His wife, Yvonne, was also taken but was released after three and a half months. Her husband was sentenced to death by the Germans, but shortly before the execution he was pardoned and at the end of September 1943 deported to the Austrian concentration camp Mauthausen. From there he was later taken to Neuengamme.

His fifty-eight-year-old colleague, Gabriel Florence, had been arrested by the German Gestapo because he was a resistance fighter in Lyon, where until March 4, 1944, he had a chair in biology. His significant scientific achievements had earned him a nomination by the French Nobel Committee. The Germans tortured him in the Gestapo prison at Montluc, near Lyon, and later brought him to Neuengamme.

A warm friendship developed between the children and the doctors. The latter were responsible for keeping the medical records for the children, and they made numerous entries on the temperature graphs by hand. Twenty years later Otto Prokop made these charts into memorials:

> With a certain sense of shock and emotion we note that the hemograms registered by the prison doctors and recorded on the temperature graphs are almost calligraphic, compared to the

other dates entered thereon. We have put these pages in the archives as a silent memorial to the victims—the inmates who were killed and the doctors and orderlies who also lost their lives.[4]

After the death of the three Polish women nurses, the two Dutch orderlies became like foster fathers to the children. The few survivors of Camp Neuengamme still speak fondly of Anton Hölzel and Dirk Deutekom.[5]

Besides taking care of the children, they were also in charge of the guinea pigs, whose cages were located in Barracks 4a. There was one guinea pig for each child, and children and animals both had the same numbers. Whenever Heissmeyer came to test the children he would also inject the guinea pigs with the same infiltrates. Scientifically, these human experiments were as worthless as those carried out on the animals. Heissmeyer would later testify in court that for him there was no difference between guinea pigs and Jewish children.

Shortly before Christmas, 1944, the children all became seriously ill. Hölzel and Deutekom tried to get some good food for them, even though they were already getting sausage and white bread daily at the request of Heissmeyer and by order of Lagerkommandant Pauly. The camp kitchen also sent over some additional food. Even the kitchen chef, SS-Oberscharführer Bladowsky, had pity on the children. "You've got children, too," Jan van Bork, a Dutch inmate, had told him, so Bladowsky even allowed the prison cooks to make some caramel candies and brown sugar cookies for the children on Christmas Eve.

On this day the solidarity of the entire camp was very obvious. Although it was strictly forbidden to enter the Heissmeyer Barracks, a number of the inmates visited the children and brought them Christmas presents—clothes that they had sewn together out of remnants. Willi Duffe, an inmate carpenter, had put together some simple wooden toys—horses, cars, a wagon, a doll in a cradle. A six-year-old Polish boy who was near-sighted received a pair of glasses that were too large for him. The starving prisoners, themselves so near death, had all sacrificed their rations—bread, margarine, marmalade—more than the children could eat. Jan van Bork even had to take back some of the food.

In mid-January, 1945, the sick children were to undergo another agony. Heissmeyer wanted to ascertain how the axillary glands had reacted to the TB infection. Since he was not a surgeon himself, he ordered a Czech inmate doctor, Dr. Bogumil Doclik, to operate on the children. In a statement given later to the British interrogation officer, Anton Walter Freud, Franzisczek Czekallá, a medical assistant from Gulcz, Poland, noted the following:

> The first aid room in Station 1 was to serve as the operating room. I was given some clamps, tweezers, scalpels, a few sharp hooks, and some Novocain. At about 7:00 p.m., when everything was ready, the orderlies brought the children from Station 4 to a private room in Station 1. I was in the first aid room of Station 1 and present at all the operations. The children were undressed down to their waists and put on the operating table. The skin under their arms was dabbed with iodine, and they were given 10 cc of 2 percent Novocain solution as a local anesthetic.
>
> Dr. Bogumil Doclik, the operating surgeon, then located the glands under the arm, made an incision 5 cm long, and took out the glands. Then he inserted cotton swabs to fill in the wound. Each operation lasted approximately fifteen minutes. On that evening nine children were treated in this manner. The French inmate doctors placed the glands into bottles with Formalin spirits and labeled these bottles with the names of the children and their numbers. After surgery the children were taken back to Station 4.
>
> A week later the children were again brought to Station 1, and I removed the swabs. At two-week intervals all the children had their glands under both arms removed. During these operations I was able to observe that many of the children had received cruciate incisions measuring 3–4 cm. What this meant I did not know.
>
> The orderly tending the children told me that the bottles with the glands were handed over to Dr. Heissmeyer. He told me further that due to poor train connections Heissmeyer waited for all the operations to be completed so that he could take all the bottles to Berlin at the same time.[6]

But he did not go to Berlin—as he had told the inmate doctors in order to keep this whole matter secret—he went to the SS sanatorium at Hohenlychen instead. There the glands were taken to the laboratory and examined histologically by Heissmeyer's colleague, Dr. Hans Klein.[7]

In the meantime, all the children had become bedridden and apathetic. They were never allowed outside but had to remain in the little rooms of the barracks with the window panes painted white. Georges Kohn was the weakest. The orderlies had to carry him to Barracks 1 for the X-rays. It was rare to hear anyone laughing in the Heissmeyer Barracks. In Birkenau the children had still romped around noisily. Here they just lay on their beds day and night, even during air raids and even as bombs fell on Hamburg and Bergedorf nearby.

The British were advancing closer and closer to Hamburg. For the fascists the end was drawing nearer. Heissmeyer conferred with SS-General Oswald Pohl about what to do with the children. Pohl himself went to Neuengamme to have a look at them.

SS-Standortarzt Dr. Alfred Trzebinski, in a statement before the British Military Tribunal, declared:

> In March, 1945, Pohl was at Camp Neuengamme together with the Kommandant of Auschwitz [Rudolf Höss]. The real purpose of Pohl's visit was to ascertain how many of the sick inmates were no longer able to work. Pauly then asked what should be done with the children. Pohl said, "I cannot make that kind of decision on my own. The Reichsführer [Himmler] would have to do that. Wait for further orders."[8]

Then came April 20, 1945. Heissmeyer had not been seen for six weeks. The British troops had occupied Harburg and were less than three miles from Hamburg. On that same day the SS in Neuengamme were celebrating the last birthday of their Führer, Adolf Hitler. It was then that the Schutzhaftlagerführer, SS-Obersturmführer Anton Thumann, came to see Trzebinski in the sickbay. He said:

> Brace yourself, I've got to tell you something not exactly pretty. An order of execution has come from Berlin. You are to kill the children by gas or by poison.

On the day that the murder of the children was being decided, Hitler was celebrating his fifty-sixth birthday in his Berlin bunker 200 miles to the east. Also present were Josef Goebbels, who eleven days later would kill his six sleeping children and then order an SS guard to shoot him; Reichsmarschall Hermann Göring, still fat despite the severe shortage of food (that night he would take off for southern

Germany by car); Foreign Minister Ribbentrop; Head of the Chancel-
lery Bormann; the architect Speer; and, above all, the three Chiefs of
Staff of the Wehrmacht—Keitel, Jodl, and Dönitz—who in the next
eighteen days would send still many thousands of soldiers to their
deaths even though they knew that this war had long since been lost.

Hitler spoke about the lovely spring at his private estate of Ober-
salzberg in the mountains. He wondered if he should fly there. Most
of those present urged him to do so. He wavered. "The situation of
the Reich isn't that bad,"[9] he said, as he drank juice while the others let
themselves be served the champagne that Himmler had provided.
The Red Army had taken Fürstenwalde, Strausberg, and Bernau,
and in the west the British were standing at the Elbe River.[10]

If the Russian advance should lead to the partition of Germany,
Grossadmiral Karl Dönitz, Commander-in-Chief of the Navy, was to
take over the command in the northern basin, Hitler ordered.
Reichsführer SS Heinrich Himmler was to remain with Dönitz, pre-
sumably to watch Dönitz or to be watched by him at this time of
betrayal.

The last person to leave was Himmler. Early that morning he had
ordered the formation of drumhead courts-martial, made up of
young, fanatical SS members who by that very evening were already
hanging soldiers and even schoolboys on lantern posts all over Berlin.[11]

Leaving Berlin, Himmler was about to embark on the greatest act
of treason imaginable for a Nazi: He went to a secret meeting with the
representative of the World Jewish Congress, Norbert Masur. This
had been arranged by Himmler's personal physician, Felix Kersten,
from Finland, a peculiar, ambivalent man who had treated Himmler
for years by "manual therapy," consisting of a combination of mas-
sage, sauna, and natural diet. In spite of his fascination with Himmler's ideas about a community of men of pure Nordic race, Felix
Kersten had become a severe critic of the concentration camp policies
of mass extermination. Surprisingly, he was nevertheless still able to
win Himmler's confidence and bring him together with Count Folke
Bernadotte of Sweden. The latter was in the end able to obtain the
release and repatriation of the Scandinavian prisoners. And so,
shortly before the blowing-up of all German concentration camps
soon to be ordered by Hitler, Kersten brought a man delegated by the
highest Jewish representative body to meet with Himmler. Kersten
tells about it:

Masur and I were the only passengers on a regularly scheduled airliner between Stockholm and Berlin. The plane was packed full with parcels sent by the Swedish Red Cross to the Red Cross in Berlin. The flight took four hours, and we saw neither Allied nor German planes in the sky. When we landed at Tempelhof Field we were greeted with a "Heil Hitler" by a police guard of five or six men standing at attention. Masur tipped his hat and said a friendly "Guten Tag." At the airport I was given the Reichsführer's safe conduct letter for Masur, signed by SS-Brigadeführer Schellenberg.[12]

From Tempelhof Kersten and Masur drove to Hartzwalde, not far from Hohenlychen. This estate had been given to Kersten as a private estate by Himmler, who in the meantime had set up his quarters there. Kersten writes:

Himmler greeted Masur with a friendly "Guten Tag" and was pleased that he had come. Then we sat down to dinner. . . . Thereupon Himmler proceeded to speak in defense of the concentration camps: They should have been called re-education camps, since they housed criminal elements besides Jews and political prisoners; in fact, because of this arrangement Germany in 1941 had been able to record the lowest crime rate in decades. True, the prisoners had to work hard, but so did all the German people. Their treatment, however, has always been just.[13]

Masur, who was very well acquainted with the existence of the extermination camps at Auschwitz, Treblinka, and Majdanek, kept quiet. And so in the end he was able to obtain from Himmler the promise of release from the Ravensbrück camp of 1,000 Jewish women, who would be picked up by Swedish Red Cross buses. Even a list of names was drawn up. Moreover, Himmler promised Masur—as he had already promised Kersten—not to evacuate any more concentration camps but to surrender them to the advancing Allied troops. The killing of Jews would stop.

At dawn they parted. Himmler drove back to Hohenlychen. Masur and Kersten left for Tempelhof and flew back as surreptitiously as they had come.

On the very day the children were to be murdered the Scandinavian prisoners were celebrating their departure from Neuengamme.

The negotiations between Himmler and Count Folke Bernadotte had been successful. The Swedish Red Cross had sent a team of doctors and nurses to Germany, together with buses, trucks, and ambulances. At first only the sick Scandinavian prisoners were permitted to leave for Sweden.

A Swedish professor, Gerhard Rundberg, was in charge of this operation. He had set up his headquarters on the private estate of the Duke of Bismarck in Friedrichsruh, in the Sachsenwald, not far from Neuengamme. Rundberg and a few other Swedish doctors were allowed to visit the Scandinavian prisoners in the sickbay barracks of Neuengamme. Here is his report:

> I looked up the Chief Physician of the camp, Dr. Trzebinski. He was a pudgy, almost bloated man, who made an unpleasant impression on most of us. We went immediately to the sickbay barracks where the Scandinavians were. In uniform and wearing boots and a cap, Dr. Trzebinski started his rounds in the most disagreeable manner I had ever experienced. He accepted or rejected our diagnoses with a nonchalant voice. He would not allow use of Latin terms for them; diagnoses were to be written down in German. "Pleuritis exsudative" (water in the lungs) became "*Feuchte Rippenfellentzündung*" ("moist inflammation of the lining of the lungs"), etc. He showed his disdain for sedimentation rates and laboratory work. He claimed one should look at patients to see what is wrong with them, and then one should judge each case by looking at the patient's legs. All the patients were asked to remove their underwear and show their legs; if these were swollen with fluid or extremely emaciated, they were accepted for transport with the notation "Overall Condition Poor." With the aid of his "diagnosis of the legs," this Nazi Party Aesculapius arrived at his decisions. As he made his pronouncements, I had to ask myself now and again if he was really a doctor.[14]

On March 31, 1945, Folke Bernadotte visited Neuengamme. He was received by Lagerkommandant Pauly. Bernadotte asked him for a tour of the camp. A Norwegian inmate, Odd Nansen, son of the Arctic explorer, Fridtjof Nansen, described the visit:

> The tour of the camp must have been a real humiliation for the Germans. They didn't say a word but could not prevent the

Swedes from talking animatedly with us and others in the various blocks. . . . They had encouraging words for everyone—words that were taken in by thousands of hungry souls and treasured in their hearts. . . . To see these SS people—the biggest tyrants in our world—to see them being treated like nothing, to see how totally superfluous and miserable they had become, this was something indescribably wonderful for us.[15]

From that day on, Neuengamme became the central collection point for all Scandinavian concentration camp prisoners leaving German camps. The white buses with the red cross and the Swedish flag went to Buchenwald, Sachsenhausen, Dachau, Ravensbrück, Neubrandenburg, Zwickau, and even Theresienstadt. From all of these camps they gathered together Scandinavian prisoners who were half starved to death. "For these tortured prisoners this was a step from hell into heaven," Jørgen H. Barfød, the Danish historian, wrote.[16]

But for the prisoners who had to remain in that hell things got worse. The Germans actually perverted the humanitarian operations of the Swedes. In order to make room for the Scandinavians, Kommandant Pauly demanded that the Swedes transfer other inmates out of Neuengamme. Colonel Björk, the military director of the Swedish operation, complied, and on March 27 and 28 the white buses under the auspices of the Red Cross took 2,000 French, Russian, and Polish inmates from Neuengamme to other camps, including the death camp at Bergen-Belsen. This was in exchange for 72 Danish concentration camp prisoners from the auxiliary camp at Hannover-Stöcken.

Professor Gerhard Rundberg, in a report to the Swedish Red Cross entitled *Rapport fra Neuengamme,* relates the following:

At this time the German authorities made further demands on the Swedish Red Cross: in exchange for reserving space in Neuengamme for all the Norwegians and Danes (who would also be provided better food), the Germans wanted the Swedish Red Cross to transport 2,000 interned foreign nationals to concentration camps in Hannover and Braunschweig.

These transports took place on March 27 and 28. According to testimony of the participating Swedes, the prisoners—French, Russian, and Polish (as well as American?)—were in very bad shape. The SS saw to it that the buses were overcrowded. Despite the protests of the Swedish drivers these helpless creatures were clubbed and kicked and, according to the same source, a number of prisoners were dead when they arrived at their destination. It was a sorry venture.[17]

A second such venture occurred on April 8, 1945. Carl Krebs, a Danish doctor, and Lieutenant Hallströhm, a Swedish driver, were to pick up ten Norwegians and one Dane from Bergen-Belsen, where in the meantime thousands of prisoners had already starved to death. The SS in Neuengamme demanded of the two that they take along a dozen "German criminals." At a stop along the way they were allowed to give the prisoners food. Dr. Krebs writes: "I was dumbfounded when I heard these prisoners whisper either 'merci' or 'spassibo,' which meant that some of these 'German prisoners' were really French, others Russian."[18]

And so a new quarter for the Scandinavians was formed in Neuengamme, separated by barbed wire from the rest of the camp. It was clean there and the inmates had comfortable beds with new mattresses; they even had Swedish showers, good clothes, and, above all, plenty to eat—while on the other side of the fence people were going hungry. Professor Rundberg describes this hunger in his report:

> After the Scandinavian camp had been mostly cleared, I went into one of the empty barracks and collected in a carton the various leftovers, such as bits of cheese, butter, sugar, bread, scraps of sausage, some honey, and whatever else I could manage to put in. I took this carton over to the barbed wire fence at a point where it was stretched double and rose six feet high, separating the Scandinavian quarter from the rest of the camp. Immediately a large number of Russians and Poles came streaming out of the nearest barracks. I began to distribute the food through the fence. They greedily stretched out their skinny, dirty hands through the barbed wire, disregarding the bloody cuts they received from the barbs. The crowd of prisoners grew like an avalanche. Then they fell to blows as the ones in the back tried to rob those who were able to snatch some crumbs. They hit, scratched, bit, and ate all at the same time. A German Lagerältester tried in vain to drive back the hungry horde with his club. He had to back off from the onslaught. Five times I filled the cartons and distributed the contents, but I had to stop before they smashed one another's heads. Blood was streaming out of noses, mouths, scratched hands, and torn ears.[19]

On April 19 all the Scandinavian transports were suddenly halted. At noon it was announced that Camp Neuengamme would be evacuated. Everyone knew what this meant: there would be death marches like those from Auschwitz. Then a new order was given: all Scandinavians, without exception, were to be taken to Denmark by the Red Cross buses.

The Swedish rescue team in Friedrichsruh had far too few vehicles for the 4,224 Scandinavian prisoners. The Danish Red Cross was asked to help. In utmost secrecy the latter had worked out a plan, to be implemented in the days after the liberation, that included the registration of all motor vehicles. The *Jyllandskorps*, an auxiliary of the Red Cross, was alerted. In a few hours ninety-four buses, eight ambulances, ten trucks, five private cars, and five motorcycles were ready and waiting in Padborg, north of the German border. All of these vehicles were quickly painted white and marked with the Red Cross and the *Danebrog*, the Danish flag. Early in the morning of April 20, six columns were heading toward Neuengamme. The Swedish Red Cross had informed the Allied forces of this transport so that they would not attack by air.

"The front was so close by now that one could not only hear the roar of the guns but also see the shells' impact in Hamburg," Jørgen Barføard writes.

> When the white buses came into the camp, they were immediately filled with prisoners and vanished again. The British aircraft made regular runs over the camp, and when the white buses stopped on the Appellplatz, the planes swooped down low and waggled their wings.[20]

At 8:00 p.m. the last five buses left Neuengamme. Dr. Roesdahl, a Danish physician, reports:

> One of my last impressions was seeing several prisoners pull one of the large carts customarily in use. On it were about six or ten pale, terribly emaciated, stiff and naked bodies with mouths open, covered only partially with some blankets. I assumed they were all dead, but suddenly one of them raised his head and for a split second looked up blankly at the many vehicles, and then fell back again. The wagon was no doubt on its way to the morgue or to the crematorium, and the fact that the man had moved would certainly not change matters in any way.[21]

Four

Everyone in Camp Neuengamme had learned of the departure of the Danes. Everyone knew that the day of liberation was now very near.

But two hours after the last Danish bus had left Neuengamme a large dark-gray truck pulled through the gates of the concentration camp. It was a mail truck, enclosed and with bars on the door in the back. SS-Unterscharführer Hans Friedrich Petersen sat at the wheel. The truck drove along the camp road and stopped in front of Barracks 4a. There it waited. It was 10:00 p.m. A half hour earlier Rapportführer Wilhelm Dreimann had gone to see the two Dutch orderlies, Dirk Deutekom and Anton Hölzel, and ordered them to wake the children and get them dressed. The two French professors, Florence and Quenouille, had to help them pack their things and take everything along. "They are being transferred to Theresienstadt." The adults, however, most likely knew what that meant; for when orderly Paul Weissmann met Gabriel Florence in passing, the latter shrugged off his consoling words, saying: "I don't believe we will see each other again." (Paul Weissmann survived the camp and later worked as Counselor at the East German Embassy in Havana.)

The children were all drowsy as Deutekom and Hölzel tried to rouse them. But when they heard that they would be taken somewhere, they quickly woke up and looked forward to going on a trip. The older ones got dressed by themselves, but Georges Kohn was so weak that the two Frenchmen had to dress him and carry him into the truck. One could look at him and see that he would not live much longer.

The children took all their things along. The smaller ones had their toys in their arms. They got into the truck. There were six prisoners in there already—Russian prisoners of war. They too were to be murdered that night. No one knows their names.

36

Later Dr. Trzebinski gave the Military Tribunal an exact description of this ride:

> That evening there was a telephone call from the SS Station. I don't know who called, because the message was received by the operator on duty. He said that I was to come to the camp, that the truck was ready. I went to the camp; the truck was at the entrance with the motor already running. I looked inside and saw twenty children sitting there as well as the four orderlies and six other men. Dreimann, Wiehagen, and Speck got into the back of the truck, and I got in front.[1]
>
> The driver had already received specific orders for departure. He drove to Spaldingstrasse. We got there in an hour. Dreimann, Wiehagen, and I got out. Speck stayed in the truck. Strippel already seemed to be waiting for us up there.[2]

SS-Obersturmführer Arnold Strippel, who had just turned thirty, commanded the auxiliary camp of the main camp of Neuengamme in the Hamburg area. He had been transferred there at the end of 1944 after a short and bloody interlude at Drütte concentration camp. Before that he had been Schutzhaftlagerführer at the Dutch camp Vught, at the very time, in fact, that the two brothers Alexander and Eduard Hornemann had been interned there. After Lagerkommandant Pauly, Strippel was the most powerful man in the camp, and he used his power brutally. He had his headquarters at 156–162 Spaldingstrasse in Hamburg. This small concentration camp housed 1,000 male prisoners—mostly Russians and Poles who were used for bomb disposal in the almost totally destroyed city of Hamburg.

> Trzebinski: "I asked Strippel to come with me into a separate room. I said, 'They've gone completely mad in Berlin. Now they've sent an order that the Heissmeyer Section has to disappear, and Pauly has thought up the pretty task for me to poison the children.' I said I couldn't do that, and anyway I had no poison with me. Strippel said, 'If Pauly ordered you to do it, you simply have to do it.' I said, 'I want to tell you something. I purposely didn't bring any poison along.' That got Strippel angry, and he said, 'So you think I'll let myself be put against the wall by Pauly if things happen here that don't suit him?' I said it was madness to kill the children. But Strippel said, 'They know

what they're doing in Berlin, and why. And if we get an order, we have to carry it out.' We continued to talk about the poison that wasn't there. Finally he said, 'If you're such a coward, I'll have to take matters into my own hands.' Then he drove his car to Bullenhuser Damm. We followed him and arrived there about ten minutes later."

At Bullenhuser Damm, in Rothenburgsort, there was a large school. It still stands today. This once lively section of Hamburg had been bombed out and was now uninhabited. The school too had taken its share of hits during the heavy bombing attack on Hamburg in July 1943. It had been burned out for the most part and had neither roof nor rafters. The Hamburg SS then took over the building, and the new life that they brought into the ruins was Death: In the fall of 1944 the first fifty concentration camp prisoners arrived there and had to put up a barbed wire fence around the area nearly ten feet high. Then they fixed up the empty building. In time more and more prisoners arrived. Since February 1945, Scandinavian prisoners had been gathered in the school; they were looked after by the Swedish Red Cross. They received food parcels, and they all had their own beds with two woolen blankets. Gregers Jensen, a Danish inmate doctor, reported:

> Bullenhuser Damm, with its 600 or so prisoners, was in many ways better than Neuengamme. We were allowed to manage the station on the second floor ourselves because the Lagerkommandant was terrified of infection and fled down the stairs as soon as there was even the slightest murmur or suspicion of typhus.

At this time the camp was under the supervision of SS-Unterscharführer Ewald Jauch. "He would go around with a club that he used for beatings and so had to get a new one almost daily," Jørgen Barfød writes.[3] Jauch's deputy was SS-Rottenführer Johann Frahm, an unusually primitive fellow who beat up his victims with whatever he happened to have in his hands.

On April 11, 1945, the Scandinavian prisoners were taken to the Neuengamme main camp, leaving the school empty. There was nothing but ruins all around.

> Trzebinski: "When we arrived and got out of the truck, Strippel, Jauch, and Frahm were just coming out the door. Strippel went right to his waiting car and said in passing that everything was in

order. I took that to mean that he arranged things in such a way as to carry out the order from Berlin. Now the occupants of the truck got out—first the Russians, then the orderlies, and then the children. The Russians were led into the boiler room; then the orderlies and the children were brought in. The orderlies were put in a room across from the children, the children themselves in an air-raid shelter. I forgot to mention that before the children and the orderlies were brought in, I had a chance to speak with Jauch. In fact, I asked him: 'Have you received any information?' He said: 'Yes, I know what's what.' I stayed with the children, for by now they had been separated from the orderlies. So I stayed with the frightened children. They had all their things with them—some food, some toys they had made themselves, etc. They sat down on the benches and were happy that they had gotten out. They didn't suspect a thing. They were between five and twelve years old—half of them boys, the other half girls. They all spoke a broken German with a Polish accent."

They waited a long time like this. Meanwhile, Jauch, Dreimann, and Frahm hanged the adults in the adjoining room. Dreimann had brought along the ropes from Neuengamme.

Jauch later admitted in court:

I knew one of the French doctors. He had treated me in Neuengamme.[4] I felt sorry for him. Dreimann had attached four ropes on a pipe about twelve feet off the ground. He put the nooses around their necks while they were standing on the floor. Dreimann pulled their feet up off the floor and held them tight for three to four minutes until they were dead. . . . As far as I could tell, these people did not put up any resistance; nor did anyone tell me that they had resisted. . . . I would have liked to save the French doctor, but I was not able to.

And so while a physician who had already murdered so many people was preparing for the murder of twenty children, two doctors met their death in this boiler room—doctors who all their lives had remained faithful to a humane ethic. Two others were hanged with them as well—Anton Hölzel and Dirk Deutekom, the "fathers" to these orphaned children. And when they were dead, it was the children's turn.

Trzebinski: "After a while Frahm came in and said the children should get undressed. I saw that the children were somewhat taken aback, so I told them: 'You have to get undressed because you'll be vaccinated against typhus.' I now took Frahm aside and asked him softly, so the children would not hear anything, 'What's to happen with the children?' Frahm was also quite pale and said, 'I'm supposed to hang the children.' I could tell stories and make myself out to be a hero, or say that I threatened him with a gun and so on, but that wouldn't be the truth. We did not discuss this any further because in my opinion the children could no longer be saved. If I had acted as a hero the children might have died a little later, but their fate could no longer be averted. I now knew what horrible end awaited them, and I at least wanted to ease their final hours. I had morphine with me in a 1 percent solution. So that I could administer the proper dosage, I diluted this bottle further with 100 grams of distilled water. Thus, depending on their ages, I could give each child the correct dosage. I went up to the door of the room where there was a stool for the syringes and another stool next to it. I called in the children one by one. They lay down over the one stool, and I gave them the shots in the buttocks, where it would be the least painful. Each child then went back into the room where they had gotten undressed, and another one came in. Frahm said the children were lying down, but that wasn't so. They lay down only afterwards, when they became tired. To make the children think that they were really being vaccinated, I used a new needle every time. According to their age and size I injected them with anywhere from 2 to 6 cubic centimeters. Out of the 120 cc about 20 cc were left over. The purpose of the individual dosages was to make the children sleepy. In the meantime they had gotten dressed again, thinking the vaccinations were over. But Frahm now told them they had to take their clothes off once more so they could be bathed. A person who has already taken part in many executions says almost automatically that the people should get undressed. And Frahm, who was rather simpleminded anyway, imagined that only people without clothes on could be hanged. I could have prevented it, but in my confusion I no longer placed any value on these things. The children started to get tired, and we laid them on the ground and covered them with their clothes. Every so often Frahm would leave the room, and I had the impression that he also took part in the execution of the men.

"I must say that in general the children's condition was very good, except for one twelve-year-old boy who was in bad shape. He therefore fell asleep very quickly. Six or eight of the children were still awake—the others were already sleeping. Now this is so terrible that it's hard for me to speak about it. But I suppose I must. Frahm lifted up the twelve-year-old boy and said to the others that he was taking him to bed. He took him to a room that was maybe six or eight yards away, and there I saw a rope already attached to a hook. Frahm put the sleeping boy into the noose and with all his weight pulled down on the body of the boy so that the noose would tighten. I had seen a lot of human suffering during my days at the camps and, in a sense, had become indifferent to it; but children being hanged—that I had never seen before. I felt sick and left the building and walked around the block a couple of times."

While Trzebinski was walking around outside feeling sick, Frahm continued the hanging of the children. At a hearing before the Military Tribunal, he denied it at first, but then admitted it:[5]

Defense Attorney Dr. Lappenberg: "What happened after the children received the injections? You said they fell asleep. Is that correct?"
Frahm: "Yes."
Lappenberg: "What happened then?"
Frahm: "Then they were put in a room."
Lappenberg: "Did you see this room?"
Frahm: "They fell asleep and did not wake up again."
Lappenberg: "How do you know that they were dead?"
Frahm: "You could see that."
Lappenberg: "What kind of shots did they receive?"
Frahm: "I don't know."
Lappenberg: "I would like to caution you once more to tell the truth. Did they die from the injection or was their death due to something else?"
Frahm: "They died from the injection. A number of them were also hanged with a rope."
Lappenberg: "When did that happen, and who hanged them?"
Frahm: "Right afterwards. Dr. Trzebinski was there and so was I."
Lappenberg: "What do you mean by right afterwards?"

Frahm: "When they were still breathing, a quarter of an hour later. I'm not exactly sure any more."

Lappenberg: "Who put the rope around the children's necks?"

Frahm: "I did."

Lappenberg: "Who gave you the order to go down to the cellar?"

Frahm: "Jauch. Oberscharführer Jauch."

Presiding judge: "Was this Jauch in charge of this work detail or was there another officer over him?"

Frahm: "He was the one responsible for this kommando. But there was another officer over him."

Presiding judge: "What is the name of this officer?"

Frahm: "Obersturmführer Strippel."

Presiding judge: "How long did the hangings of the children go on?"

Frahm: "About ten minutes."

Presiding judge: "In your opinion, were the children very ill? Were they lying down, or were they healthy?"

Frahm: "They were sick; most of them were lying down."

Presiding judge: "Were the children able to walk?"

Frahm: "Yes."

Presiding judge: "Who brought each of the children into the room where they were to be injected?"

Frahm: "They were called in."

Presiding judge: "And every child came?"

Frahm: "Yes. Some of them were also brought in."

Presiding judge: "Who brought them in?"

Frahm: "I brought them in, too."

Presiding judge: "Were the children naked?"

Frahm: "They were undressed."

Presiding judge: "Where were they undressed?"

Frahm: "In the room where they were waiting."

Presiding judge: "Did the children cry?"

Frahm: "No."

Presiding judge: "Only the children who were still breathing were hanged?"

Frahm: "Yes."

Presiding judge: "About ten of them?"

Frahm: "I don't know for sure any more."

Presiding judge: "And one child after another was hanged or a few at a time?"

Frahm: "Two at a time."

Presiding judge: "So you mean to say two of them were pulled up over the pipe at one time?"

Frahm: "The grown-ups were pulled up over the pipes. The children were hanged on the hooks."

Presiding judge: "How many children were hanged at one time on these hooks?"

Frahm: "One."

Presiding judge: "Not two?"

Frahm: "There were two hooks there."

Defense Attorney Dr. Halben: "And while this was going on in the cellar, did you also see Obersturmführer Strippel?"

Frahm: "Yes, he was there, too."

Presiding judge: "Did you hear that afterwards the SS were given remuneration, as well as cigarettes and liquor?"

Frahm: "We got a few cigarettes. And some whiskey."

Presiding judge: "Who all got cigarettes and whiskey?"

Frahm: "Oberscharführer Jauch and I."

Presiding judge: "Did no one speak to you after all this was over?"

Frahm: "I don't know."

Trzebinski also did not speak when he came back in. The murder of the children was not yet completed.

Trzebinski: "Some of them were already gone. A few were not yet sleeping, and they asked me, 'Are we going to be put to bed soon, too?' I went into the room where the first hanging had taken place and noticed that on another hook on the wall a girl was hanging. In a closet next to the room the bodies of three children were lying, among them that of the boy who had been hanged first."

Trzebinski gave the six children who were still awake a second injection of morphine. Then he waited until they were all asleep and left—on foot, to Spaldingstrasse, to fill out the medical records. But he was not able to do this properly, he said, because "my thoughts were constantly at Bullenhuser Damm."

There, in the meantime, the mail truck had driven up a second time. It brought a new load of prisoners—Russians. One knows neither their names nor exactly how many there were. "About twenty-five," Unterscharführer Speck told the British Military Tribunal. They had been picked up at the Spaldingstrasse concentration camp—Strippel's headquarters. Jauch and Frahm brought them out of the truck in groups of four and led them down to the cellar of the school. There they were hanged just like the first group of Russians, the orderlies, and the doctors. Speck stayed outside by the truck during this time, as did Petersen, the driver. When eight Russians had been murdered and the third group of four was about to be taken off the truck, the Russians suddenly all jumped off, threw salt into the faces of the SS, and tried to flee.

> Speck: "They came out shouting, and I felt a handful of salt fly in my face. I got into a scuffle with one of the prisoners and used my gun to shoot him down. I had to do it in self-defense."

At least three of the imprisoned Soviet soldiers were shot by Speck while trying to escape. Some succeeded in their flight, six of them, it seems. Whether they got back home to Russia alive, no one knows.

By then it was already light outside. Trzebinski went back into the school. As a physician he had to carry out a formality: to confirm the death of the prisoners.

> Trzebinski: "I now went into the building to see about the children. There was no one in the room where they had been. Only some of their belongings were lying there. I went to the room where the hangings had taken place and found it locked. I took the matter up with Frahm, and he opened the room for me. All the children were lying there, and they all had rope marks around their necks. I examined each child to see if it was indeed dead. Then I went into the room where the hanged men were and examined them as well to see if they were dead. And so this sad chapter was closed. Then we drove back. I never again spoke another word to any of the people who had been at Bullenhuser Damm. I didn't feel like it."

That is not completely true. For Jauch can be believed when he testified that after the murder of the children the first thing Trzebinski did was to ask for a cup of strong coffee, which he drank in his—Jauch's—room. After that he ordered Frahm to burn the children's clothing in the coal stove in the bathroom. Then the truck returned to Neuengamme. Dreimann and Speck sat in the back; Petersen, the driver, and Trzebinski, the doctor, sat in front. Jauch and Frahm stayed at Bullenhuser Damm and locked up the corpses. Then they got some sleep. This was between 6:00 and 6:30 in the morning of April 21, 1945.

While the children and the adults were being hanged, there was a man present, somewhere on the ground floor, the only civilian with access to this concentration camp—the janitor, Wilhelm Wede. He said later that he heard nothing of what was going on that night. He said he was sleeping. In the morning when he went to look after the heating, he threw into the furnace whatever was lying around. Some wooden toys and a couple of old dolls.

The children were dead now, but their corpses were locked up in a room in the cellar of the school at Bullenhuser Damm. If the British were to find them, they would have cause for an even stronger accusation: their bodies bore not only the wounds caused by the medical testing but also the marks of hanging.

Clearly Lagerkommandant Max Pauly had not previously given any thought to how to dispose of the dead victims. When on April 20 SS-Unterscharführer Ewald Jauch telephoned his superior from Bullenhuser Damm and asked what should be done with the children's corpses, the Kommandant was evasive. "Pauly ordered me to keep the corpses at Bullenhuser Damm until further orders arrived," Jauch declared before the British Military Tribunal. "I pointed out that it was impossible to keep them in the cellar. But he insisted that no decision had as yet been made about where the corpses should be taken."

When night had come again—the night of April 21–22, 1945— the same mail truck that had brought the children to Hamburg for their execution arrived again at Bullenhuser Damm. Jauch reported at the trial:

> The bodies were taken by truck from Bullenhuser Damm to Neuengamme. Strippel came with the truck, and I took him and the other people who had come with him down to the cellar and showed them where the corpses were. The next day Pauly called up and complained because I had turned the bodies over to Strippel without orders. He threatened to have me court-

martialed. Pauly was annoyed that the bodies had been taken back to Neuengamme. I think he was annoyed because of the possibility of someone or other finding out about the whole matter.

SS-Unterscharführer Wilhelm Brake, director of the crematorium at Neuengamme concentration camp, had the bodies of the twenty dead children and twenty-eight adults cremated during the night of April 21, 1945.

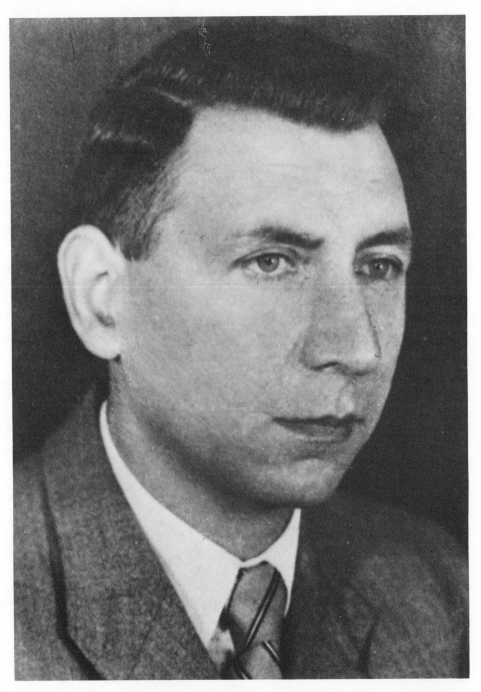

Dr. Kurt Heissmeyer came from a Nazi doctor's family. His animosity
toward Jews was influenced by his membership in a Marburg fraternity called "Arminia." He considered concentration camp inmates
inferior human beings, on whom he could experiment as if they
were guinea pigs.

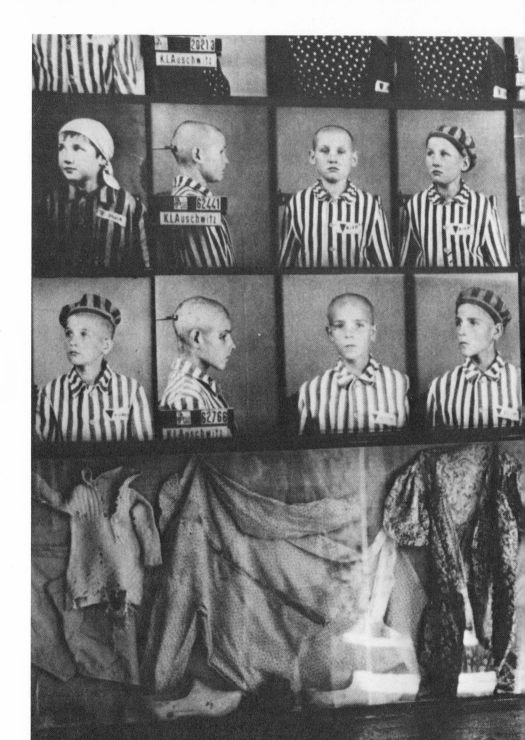

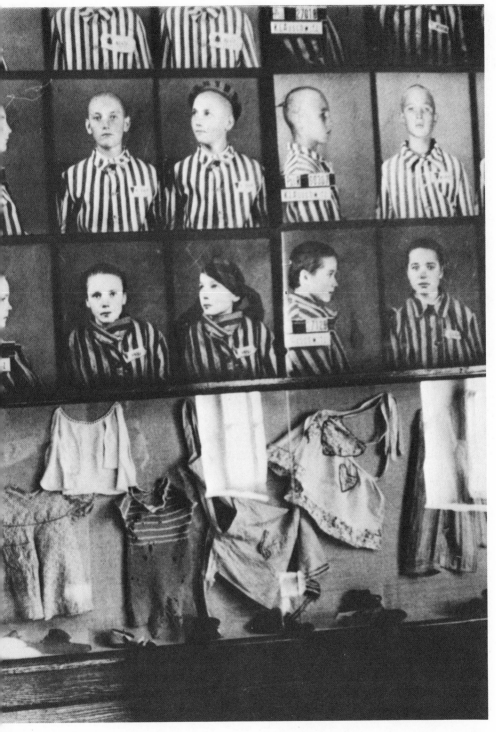

A wall of exhibits in today's Auschwitz Museum shows what remained of the murdered children: some file photos and a few pieces of clothing.

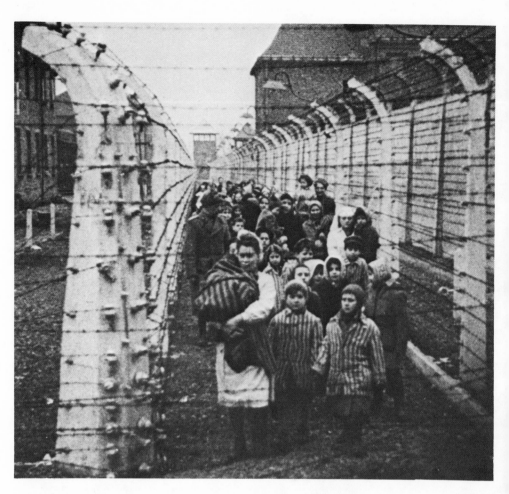

When the Red Army
liberated Auschwitz on
January 27, 1945, there
were only three-hundred
children left alive.

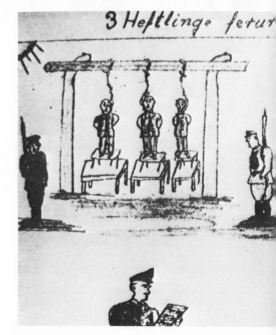

3 Heftlinge ferur

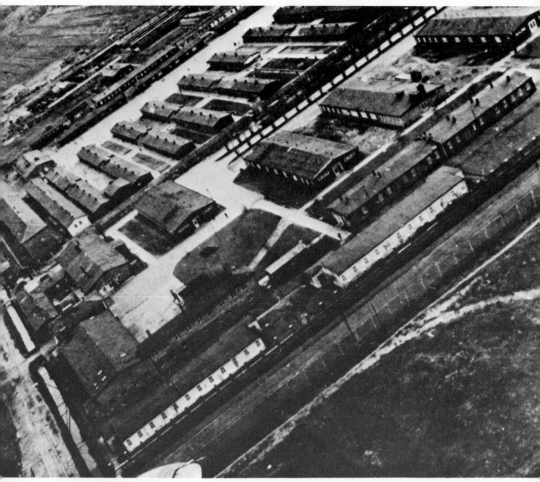

A British aereal photograph of Neuengamme concentration camp near Hamburg.

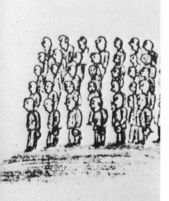

zum Galgen

This is how an unknown child in Theresienstadt portrayed daily life in that concentration camp. (The caption at the top of the drawing reads "3 prisoners sentenced to hang.")

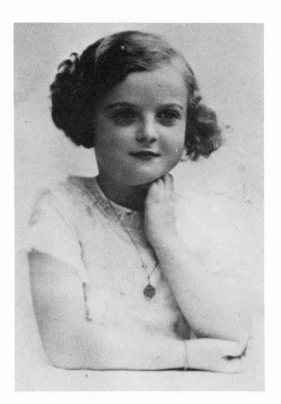

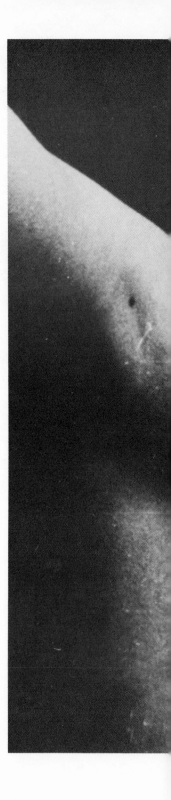

Jacqueline Morgenstern, as a seven-
year-old in Paris. And as a twelve-
year-old in Neuengamme concentration camp.

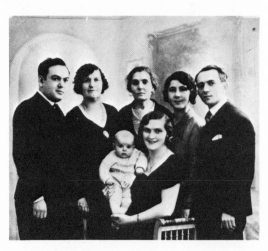

Jacqueline Morgenstern on the lap of
her mother Suzanne. From left to
right, her father, her two grand-
mothers, her Aunt Dorothéa
Morgenstern with her husband
Leopold.

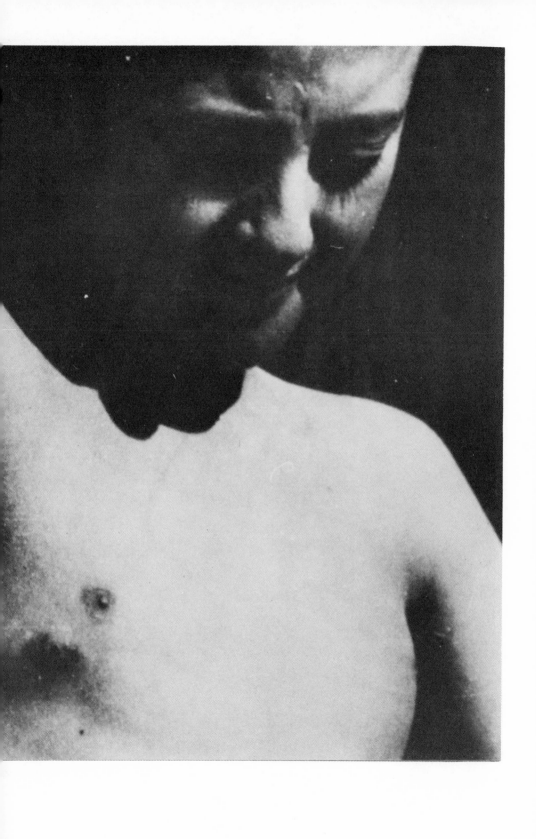

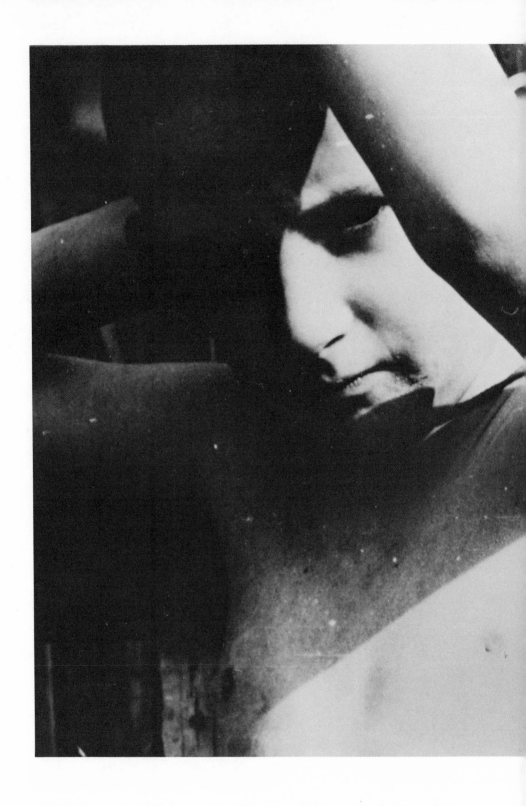

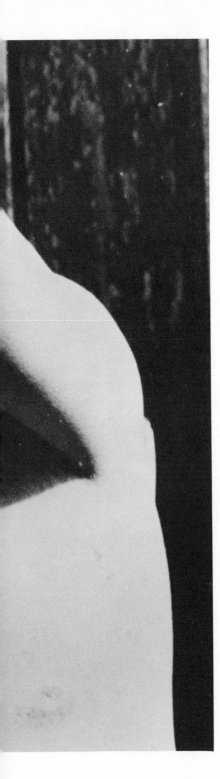

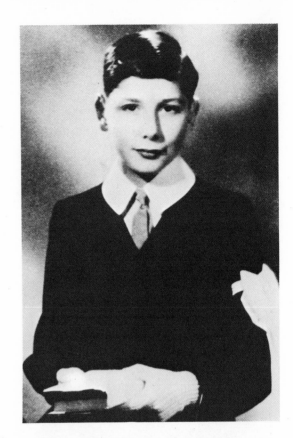

Georges Kohn, as a ten-year-old at his first communion in Paris. And as a twelve-year-old in Neuengamme concentration camp.

Georges Kohn, two years
old, in the arms of his
mother. The Kohns were
a well-to-do and happy
family in Paris before the
Nazis came. The mother
starved to death in
Bergen-Belsen.

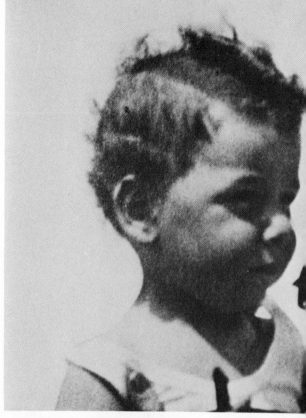

Georges Kohn, seven
years old, with his sister
Rose-Marie, his brother
Philippe, and his sister
Antoinette, who perished
with her mother in
Bergen-Belsen.

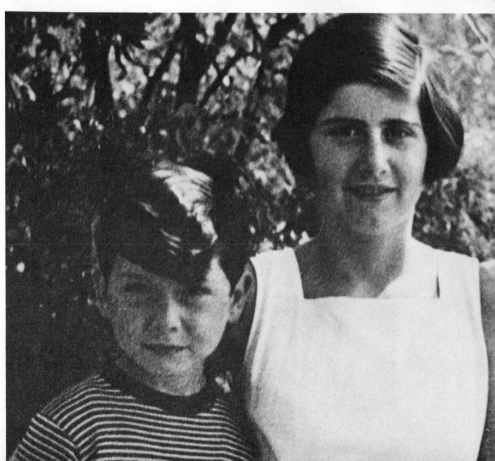

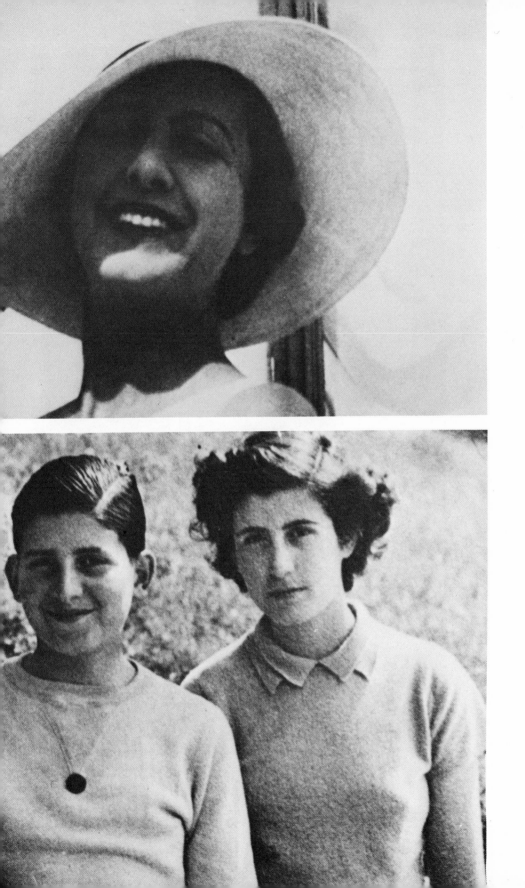

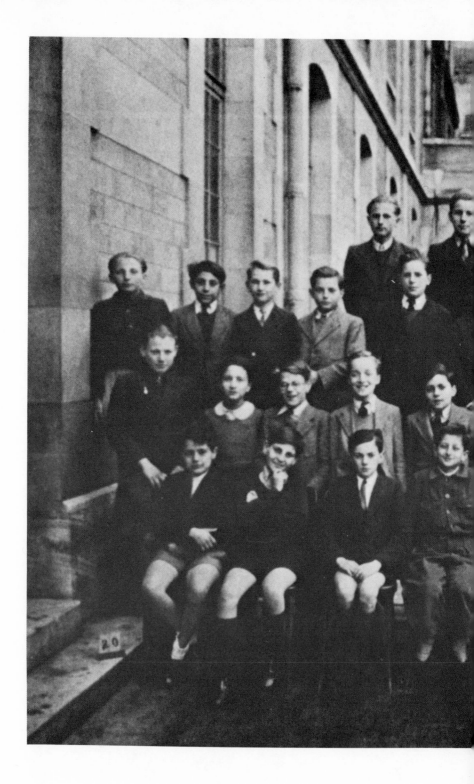

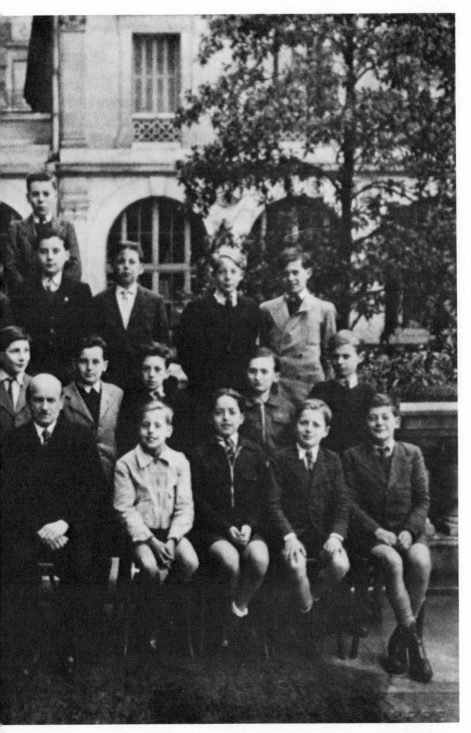

This group photo of Georges Kohn's class
was taken shortly before the deportation of
the Kohn family and the liberation of Paris:
Georges Kohn is seated behind his teacher
to the left.

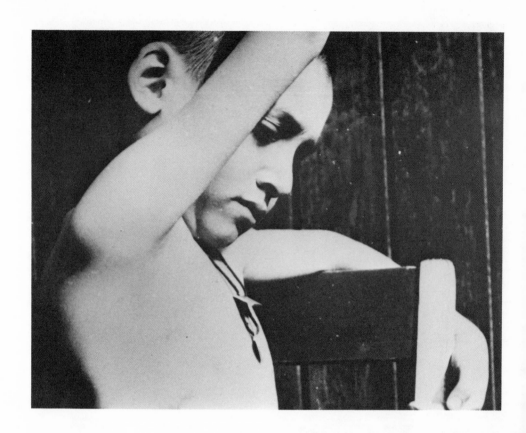

Eduard and Alexander
Hornemann in Neuen-
gamme concentration camp.
And with their mother.
Elisabeth Hornemann, who
died of typhoid fever in
Auschwitz at age thirty-seven.

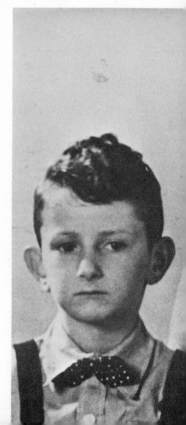

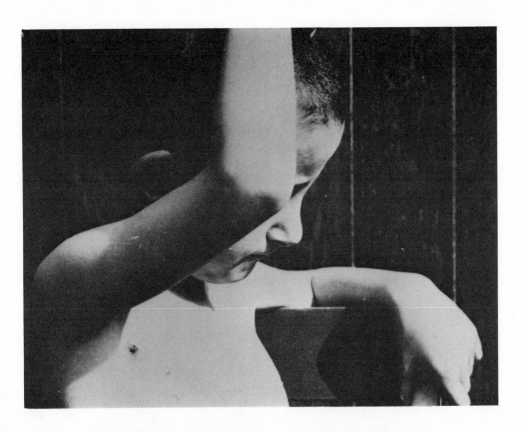

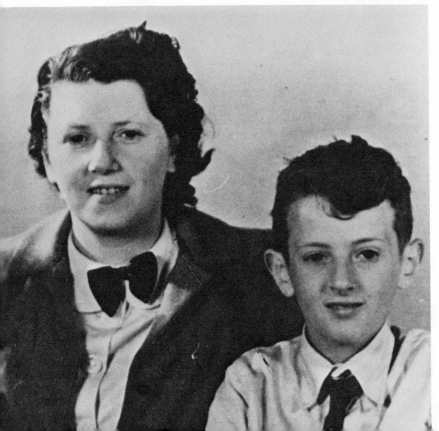

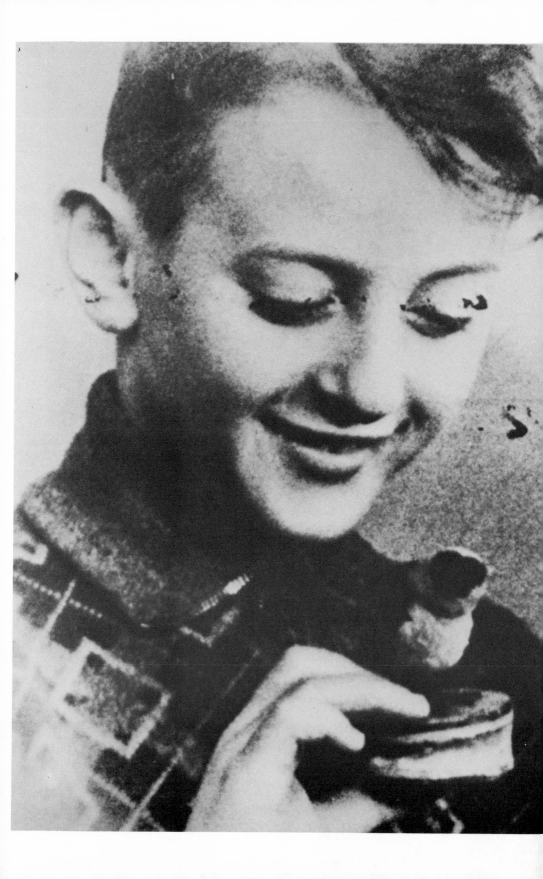

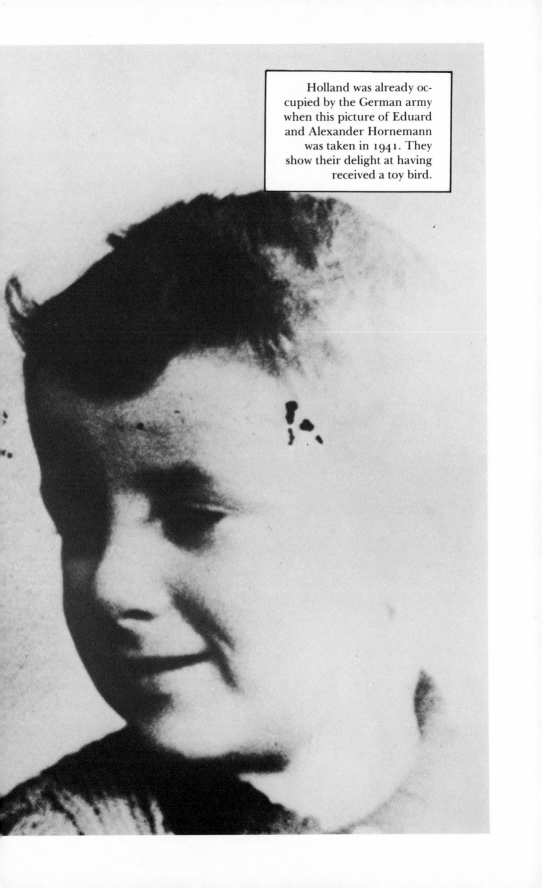

Holland was already oc-
cupied by the German army
when this picture of Eduard
and Alexander Hornemann
was taken in 1941. They
show their delight at having
received a toy bird.

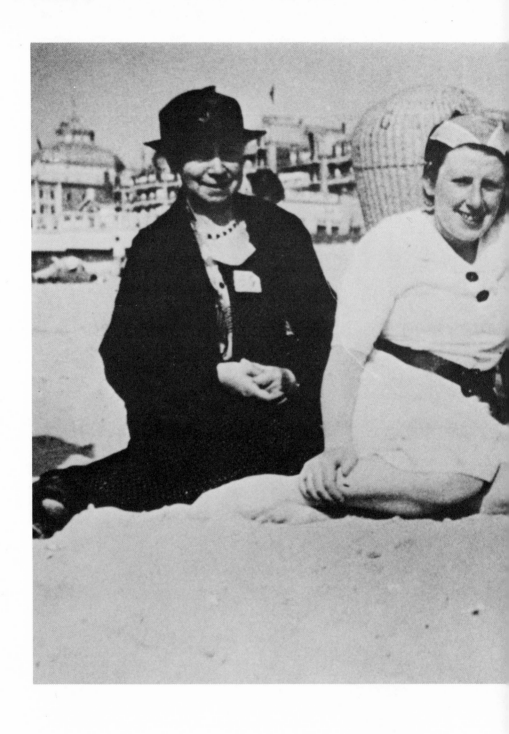

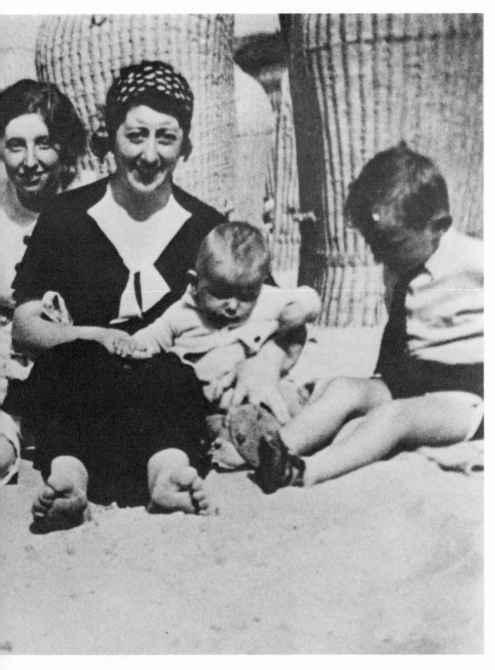

A peaceful family scene on the peaceful
beach of Scheveningen in 1938: Grandmother Hornemann and mother Elisabeth
with her housekeeper Gien de Haas and
Tante "Ans" playing with "Lexje" and
"Edo." "Ans" escaped deportation by hiding
for months in a convent.

After the lymph glands under their arms had been removed, the twenty children were photographed by SS photographer Josef Schmidt. Heissmeyer took these photos with him to Hohen-lychen and hid them in a tin box. Nineteen years after the end of the war, the buried box was found again. The films were still usable.

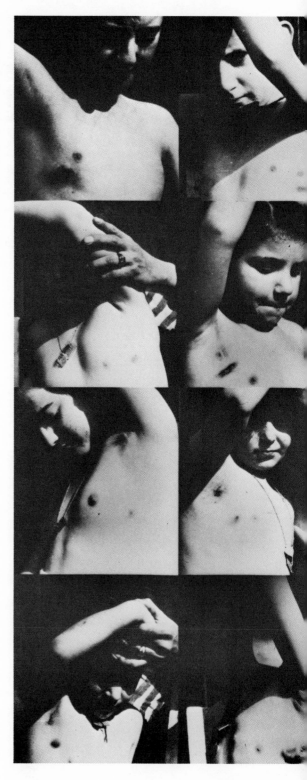

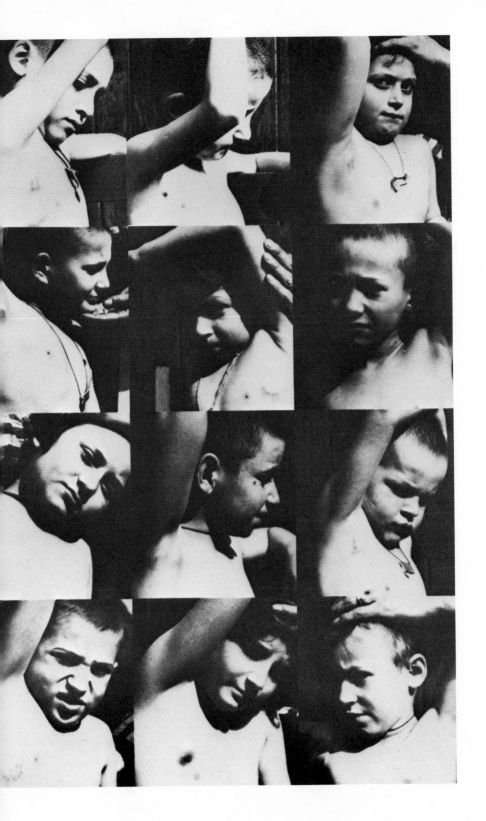

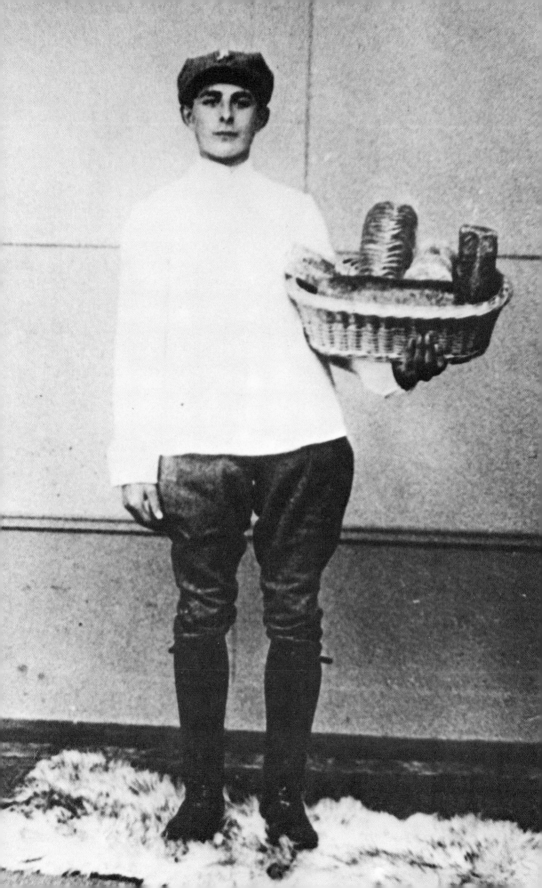

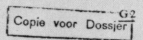

G2

Sterbeurkunde

(Standesamt Hamburg-Neuengamme – – – – – Nr. 46/1948)

Der Fahrer Antonie H ö l z e l – – – – – – – – –

– – – – – – – – – – – – – – –,Religion unbekannt–

ohnhaft in 's-Gravenhage – – – – – – – – – – – –

ist am 20.April 1945 – – – – – um –24– Uhr –00– Minuten

in Hamburg, Schule am Bullenhuser Damm – – verstorben.

Der Verstorbene war geboren am 7. Mai 1909 – – – –

in Deventer , Holland – – – – – – – – – – – – – –

– –

D er Verstorbene war — nicht — verheiratet (Namen der –

Ehefrau unbekannt) – – – – – – – – – – – – – –

– –

Hamburg, den 18. März 1950

Der Standesbeamte
In Vertretung

(Buck)

(Siegel)

Todesursache: Erhängen.

Carstensen & Plombeck, EP 260, Hbg.-Altona 667. 6000 1. 50. A.

Dutch orderly Anton Hölzel, arrested for distributing Communist newspapers, was hanged on April 20, 1945, together with the children. The document on the right is his death certificate.

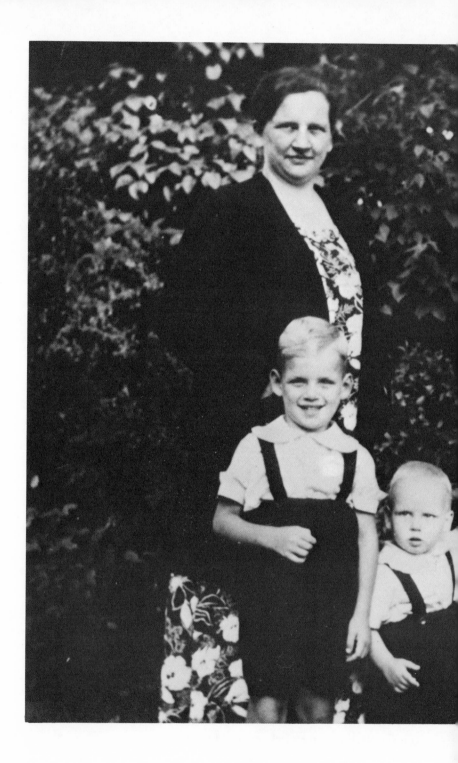

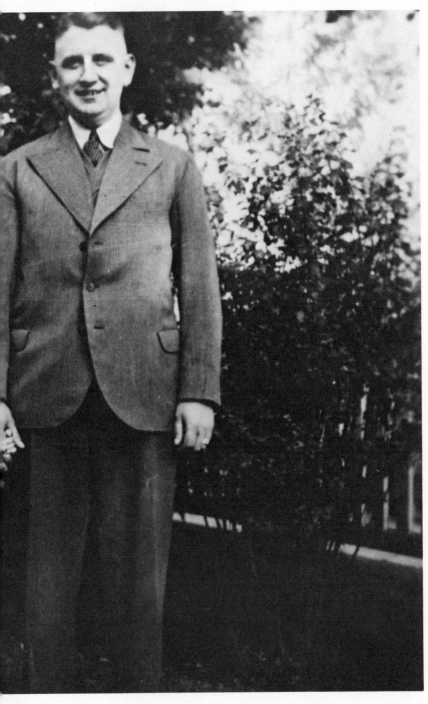

A German family: concentration camp
Kommandant Max Pauly with his wife
Käthe and his two children, Hans-Werner
and Dieter, in the garden of his home in
Danzig-Adlershorst. Hans-Werner remembers still today Hitler's visit to Danzig: "Hitler shook my hand."

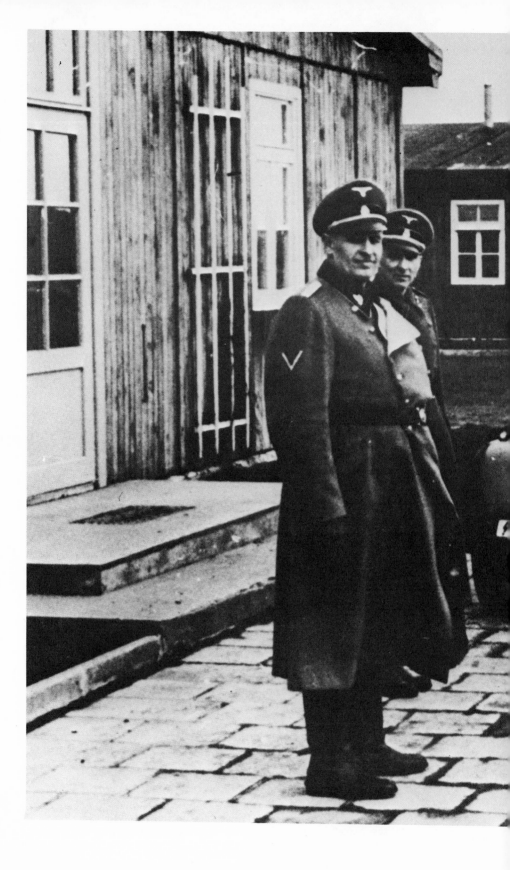

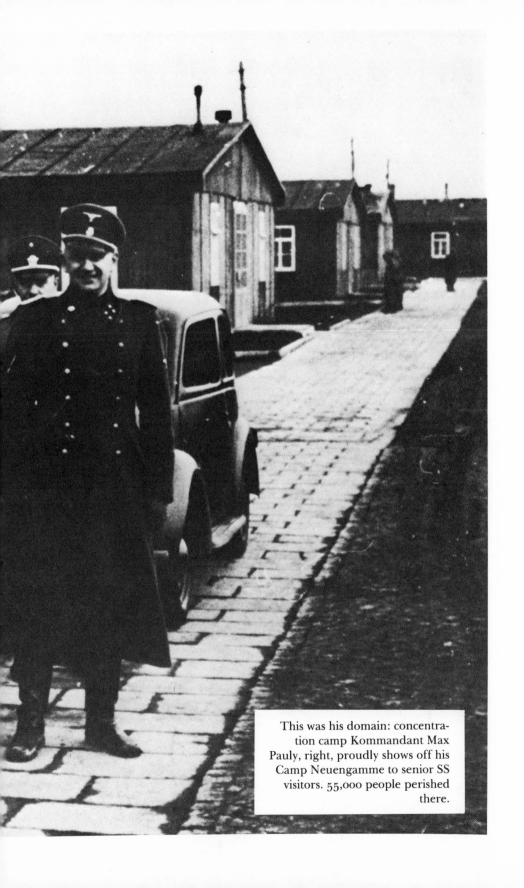

This was his domain: concentration camp Kommandant Max Pauly, right, proudly shows off his Camp Neuengamme to senior SS visitors. 55,000 people perished there.

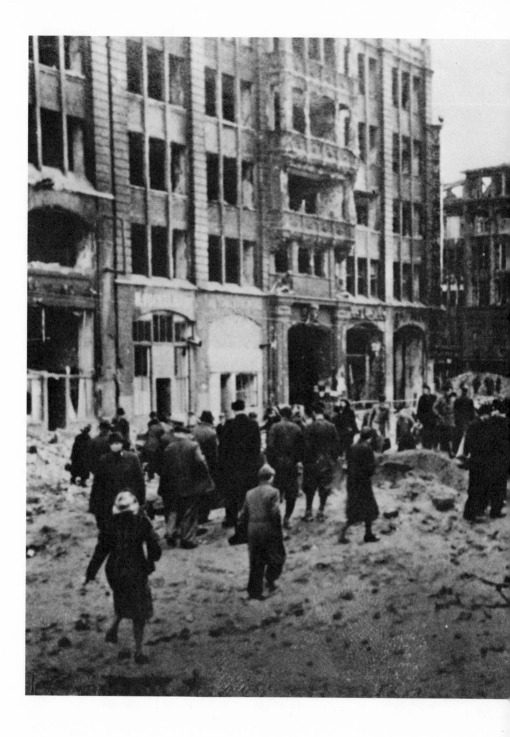

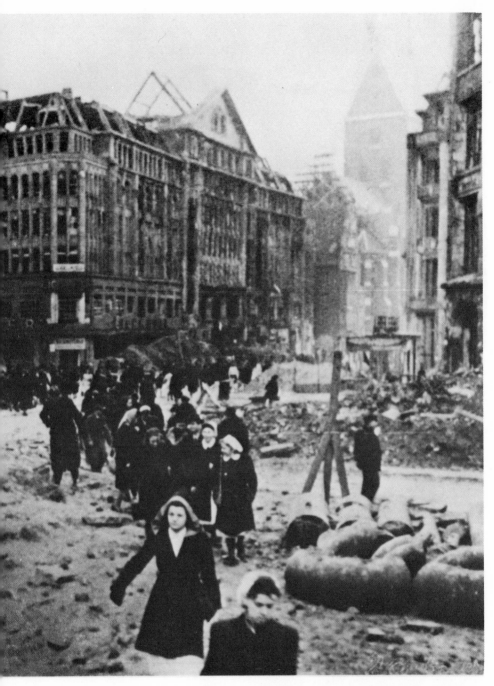

April 20, 1945, on Mönckebergstrasse in
the bombed-out city of Hamburg. Not far
from here the twenty children were hanged
on the evening of this same day.

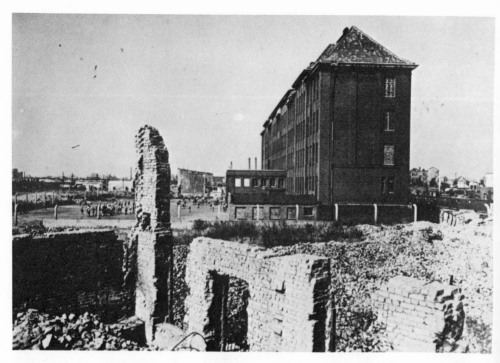

The school on Bul-
lenhuser Dam in Ham-
burg. During the war it
was an auxiliary camp of
Neuengamme concentra-
tion camp. Today it is
once more a school.

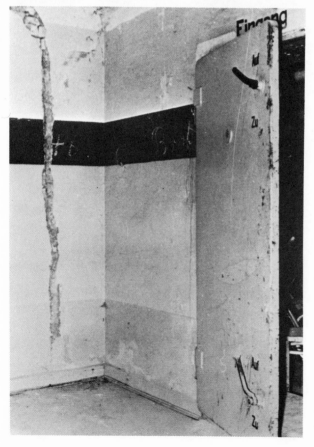

This is the murder site: in
the air raid shelter of the
school twenty Jewish children and twenty-eight
adults were hanged on
April 20, 1945.

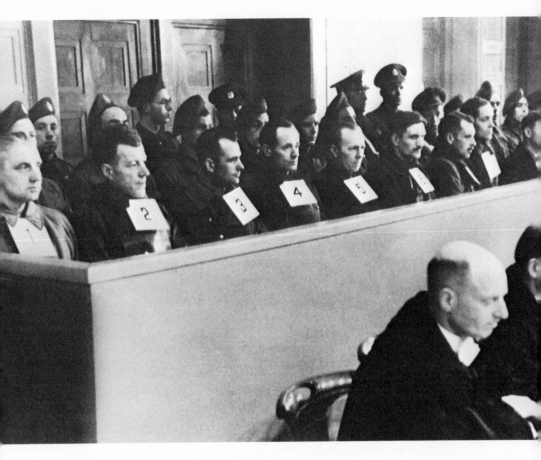

In 1946 the criminals of Neuengamme were
sentenced to death at the Curiohaus trial.

No. 1—Lagerkommandant Max Pauly.
No. 3—Schutzhaftlagerführer Thumann.
No. 5—SS-Unterscharführer Wilhelm
Dreimann. Below, right—Dr. Wessig,
Pauly's defense attorney.

ihr guten Willens seid, dieses
zu verhindern.
Es hätte zwar nichts genützt, aber mein
Gewissen wäre entlastet worden, wenn
es mich auch mein eigenes Leben
gekostet hätte.
Ich kann mir keinen Vorwurf machen,
dass ich den Kindern vor ihrer Hin-
richtung eine barmherzige Morphin-
spritze gemacht habe. Dies war
im Gegenteil eine humane Tat,
die ich mich nicht zu schämen
brauche.
Ich bin bereit, diesen gesamten Vor-
gang zu beschwören.

Hamburg, d. 24. März 1946

Dr. Alfred Trzebinski

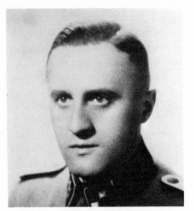

Alfred Trzebinski, a physician and SS-Hauptsturmführer, declared in written notes for his testimony that the morphine injections for the children had been a humane act.

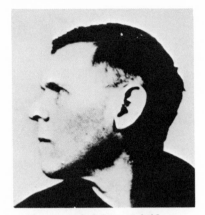

Kommandoführer Adolf Speck guarded the children's transport.

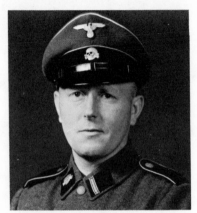

Unterscharführer Wilhelm Dreimann brought the children down into the cellar.

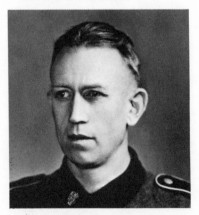

Rottenführer Johann Frahm put the rope around the children's necks.

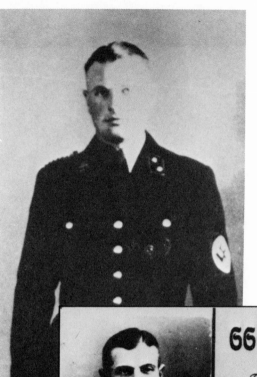

SS-Obersturmführer Arnold Strippel began his career in the concentration camps as a guard in Sachsenburg concentration camp. Thereafter he worked in many other camps between Natzweiler and Majdanek and left a bloody trail through Europe. He was pardoned and granted 121,500 marks in compensation for time spent in prison. Today Strippel lives in Frankfurt.

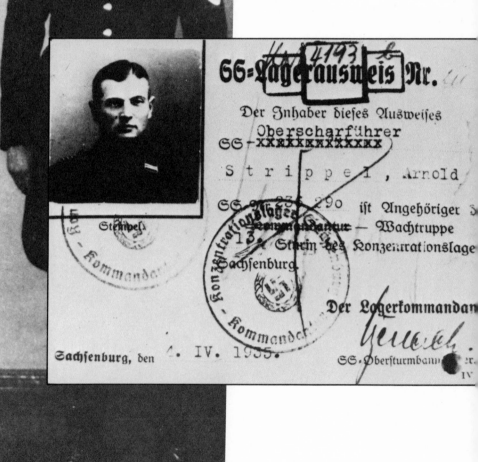

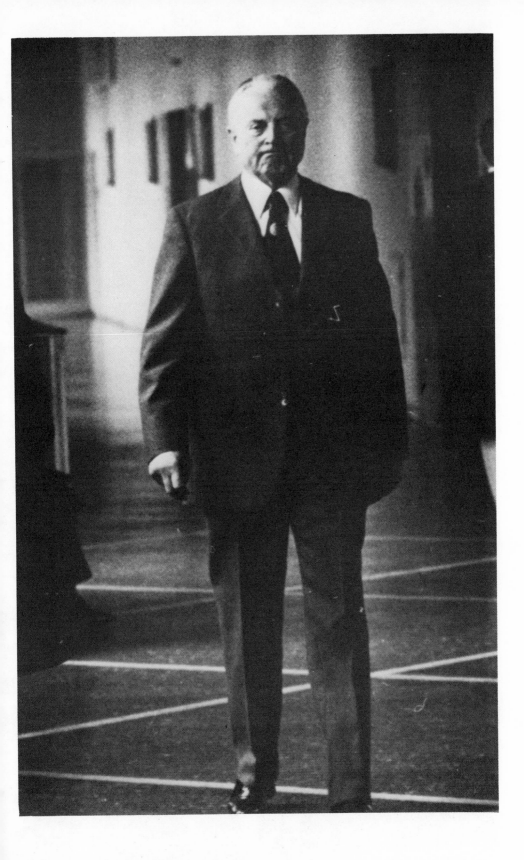

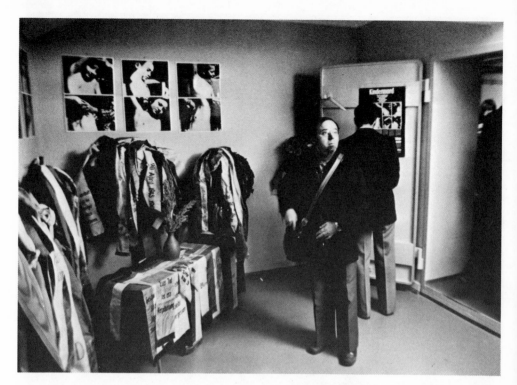

On April 20, 1979, Henri
Morgenstern, from Paris,
stood for the first time in
the cellar of the Bullen-
huser Damm School,
where his cousin Jac-
queline had been hanged.

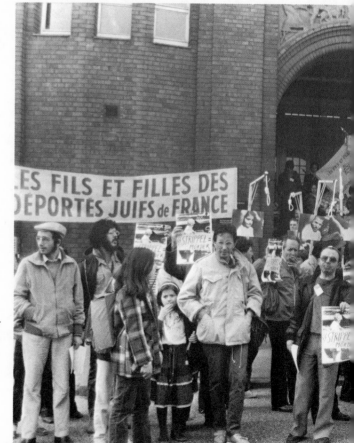

French Jews in front of
the school at Bullenhuser
Damm, April 20, 1982.
Henri Morgenstern, cen-
ter, holding poster.

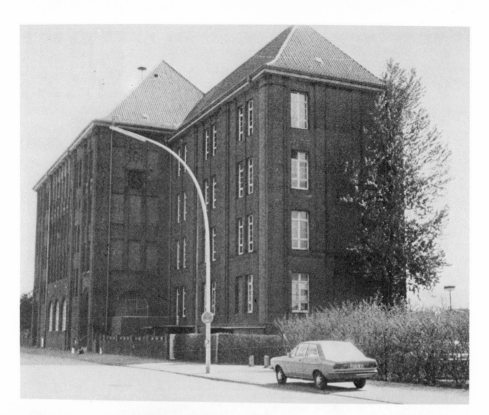

The school at Bullenhuser Damm has been renamed the Janusz Korczak School. Korczak, a Polish-Jewish physician and writer, was murdered in Treblinka with a group of Jewish orphans he had attended and tried to protect.

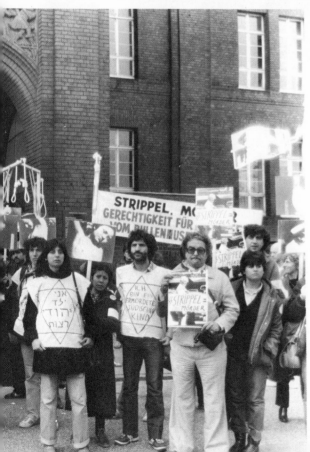

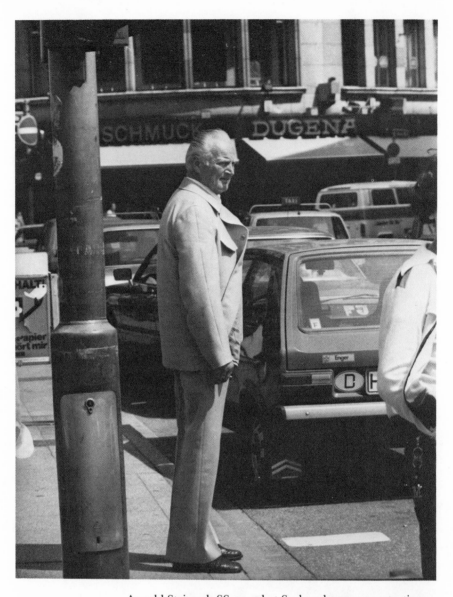

Arnold Strippel: SS guard at Sachsenburg concentration camp in Saxony in 1934; Rapportführer at Buchenwald in 1938; SS-Stabscharführer at Natzweiler concentration camp in Alsace in 1940; Untersturmführer at Majdanek concentration camp in Poland in 1942. He continued his SS career with tours of duty at Ravensbrück concentration camp, the labor camp Peenemünde, Vught concentration camp in Holland, the labor camp Drütte near Braunschweig, and the auxiliary camp Dessauer Ufer in Hamburg Harbor. As SS-Obersturmführer, he assumed command of all the Hamburg auxiliary camps of Neuengamme concentration camp, including the camp in the school at Bullenhuser Damm, and was acting in that capacity in April 1945 when the children were murdered.

Five

The Neuengamme concentration camp was coming to its end, as indeed was the entire German Reich. In seven years more than 40,000 people had been killed in Neuengamme, but 10,000 prisoners were still alive—witnesses to the crimes. They, too, were to be destroyed—drowned in the waters of Lübeck Bay.

Heinrich Himmler, the "Reichsführer SS," ordered Count Bassewitz-Behr, Senior SS Officer and Chief of Police of Hamburg, to have the Neuengamme prisoners taken to Lübeck. From there they were to be loaded onto the last ships still remaining in Nazi hands. Karl Kaufmann, Gauleiter and Reichsstatthalter in Hamburg, as well as the person in charge of marine affairs, requisitioned the two ships: the *Cap Arcona*, from the Hamburg–South American Steamship Agency (which had formerly used it as a luxury liner), and the freighter *Thielbeck*, from the shipping company Knöhr and Burchard, also of Hamburg.

The evacuation of Neuengamme surprised both the prisoners and a clandestine committee of prisoners, led by a very active Belgian lawyer, André Mandrycks. An armed uprising was being prepared. Wassilij Bukrejew, a Soviet major, headed the five-member military committee that had established three prisoner battalions. Twenty-one rifles lay hidden in the "Metal Works," three pistols elsewhere in the camp. The assault on the SS barracks and its 800-man guard had been planned in detail. But the uprising was to take place only after the rebellious prisoners had succeeded in establishing contact with the British.

This military committee met on April 18, 1945. One of its members, Bogumil Doclik, a Czech doctor who had been forced to remove the lymph nodes from the children, noted in his diary:

> It was a rough-and-tumble meeting. The Russians insisted on taking over power by force of arms. If we didn't rise up as soon as

possible and use to our advantage this moment of indecision on the part of the camp's leadership, we would condemn the entire camp to death.[1]

But the majority felt it was still too early to revolt. Thus, by their indecision the prisoners lost their last chance for freedom. For now the transports began. Their organization was torn apart. The whole camp was condemned to death. The prisoners were taken in batches to Lübeck in container cars. Hundreds died on the way from exhaustion and weakness.

The small freighter *Athens* brought the prisoners to the *Cap Arcona,* which was anchored near Neustadt in Lübeck Bay. It had engine trouble and was nearly out of fuel. Her captain, Heinrich Bertram, was a brave man. He refused to take the prisoners on board. The *Athens* had to return with them to Lübeck. Bertram later spoke the following for the record:

> I didn't think twice about refusing to take the prisoners on board. For every responsible seaman knows that, given the tremendous risks at sea in a modern war, it would be irresponsible to take on people in such huge numbers unless transporting them by sea was absolutely necessary.[2]

For days the captain stuck to his refusal. Twice the *Athens* had to turn back with its cargo of 2,300 prisoners and 280 SS guards. On April 26, SS-Sturmbannführer Gehrig, the administrative head of Neuengamme concentration camp, went out to the *Cap Arcona* with an SS-Kommando and threatened Captain Bertram with arrest if he continued to refuse to take the prisoners on board. He said he had an arrest warrant with him. Captain Bertram capitulated:

> I now realized that not even my own death would prevent the prisoners being loaded on board, and so I told the SS officer that as of this moment I was, as a matter of principle, relinquishing all responsibility for my ship.[3]

The loading of the prisoners began. So that no one could escape, SS-Obersturmführer Klebeck, together with Unterscharführer Tümmel, had gathered up all the life jackets and locked them up.

On April 30 there were nearly 10,000 prisoners on the three ships now anchored in Lübeck Bay: 4,600 on the *Cap Arcona,* 1,998 on the *Athens,* and 2,800 on the *Thielbeck.* They were extremely tense, for they sensed that they had been concentrated on these ships in order to be murdered. Death could come either by way of torpedoes from German submarines or by explosives laid in the ships themselves. However, it turned out to be bombs and bullets from British planes that would kill most of them—Himmler had presented these overloaded ships as targets to the British.

On May 3, 1945, at 12:30 p.m., Captain Nobmann of the *Athens* received a dispatch on the wireless from the Standortkommandant of Neustadt ordering him to come into port and take on additional prisoners. The ship docked at 1:45 p.m. at the Neustadt pier.

Forty-five minutes later, at 2:30 p.m., there began the biggest catastrophe at sea of World War II. A squadron of British fighter bombers flew over Lübeck Bay. Several of them attacked the *Athens*, which responded with antiaircraft fire. Three small bombs hit the ship. Firing ceased and the white flag was raised. The 1,998 prisoners jumped on land and were saved.

Then the planes flew over the other two ships. Witnesses report that the prisoners on deck waved at the aircraft with their caps and white scarves. They shouted with joy: "Freiheit!" "Liberté!" "Wolnosc!"

But the British fired sixty-four rockets at the *Cap Arcona,* and in a second wave their planes dropped sixteen heavy bombs. Only one missed its target. The others hit the overloaded ship, lifted it up, and transformed it into a blazing sea of fire. Then yet another wave attacked the *Thielbeck,* which sank in minutes.

Of the 2,800 prisoners on the *Thielbeck,* 50 were saved. The others were killed by the bombs and the strafing or were crushed by the shifting deckload or drowned in the ice-cold water. For the 2,000 prisoners below deck it was impossible even to come up. "Just as one of them reached the edge of the deck he was pulled down by the others, who hung on him like grapes, and the ship, already filled with water, took her victims down with her into the depths," reports one of the few survivors.[4]

About 3:30 p.m., the ship sank. Approximately 2,750 prisoners, some guards and crew members, and Captain John Jacobsen went down with it.

Of the more than 5,000 prisoners on the *Cap Arcona,* about 350 were able to save themselves. Therefore only a small part of the terrible events on board the burning ship became known. On D-Deck 700 gravely ill and dying men burned to death. In the banana coolers, deep inside the ship, the SS had put Russian prisoners of war. Only a very few of them were able to come up safely to the top; the others suffocated or died in the flames. Among those who died was André Mandrycks, the political head of the committee of prisoners.

In the stairwells of the ship many hundreds of people tried to push themselves upward. But then the burning deckhead crashed down and buried them. Two French prisoners, named Langlet and Fougassier, tried to save a Belgian who had lost both legs, torn off by bomb fragments. They carried him up to the top deck on the remains of a door. As they were looking for something with which to bandage his wounds, panic broke out, and he burned to death with many others.

Most of the SS men were able to jump overboard. They had taken the life jackets out of their locked compartments. Some of them even tried to hold back the prisoners at gunpoint as they were pushing to get out. Heinrich Mehringer and Aleksander Machnew, two of the prisoners, saw an SS man with two guns in his hands shooting at the prisoners and trying to close off the stairway leading to the deck. When he had used up all the bullets, he was knocked down and trampled to death by the onrushing mob.[5]

Other SS men were beaten to death with iron bars or clubs; among them, SS-Unterscharführer Heinrich Wiehagen, one of the murderers of Bullenhuser Damm.

Heinrich Mehringer, a prisoner who survived, describes how he was able to save himself:

> My back and my head were already burning, yet I didn't feel the fire as hot but cold because I was so agitated. Just then, at the last possible moment and at the greatest of risks, I saw an iron pipe above me that was used in putting up awnings. I was just barely able to reach up and grab it with one arm and with superhuman effort to pull myself up. Thus I came to stand on the heads of the thronging mass of men. About ten others were lucky enough to follow me before the flames sealed the rest into one great fiery heap. We literally ran for our lives on the heads of our fellow prisoners as on a pavement. When we got to the railing we quickly climbed outboard, down to the small deck where the rowboats were. . . . On the deck above us all our comrades burned to death. After a while the fire had nothing more to feed on.

There was a dead silence. As soon as we could we looked to see what had happened. It was a horrible sight: more than 200 burned and charred bodies welded together in a single clump.[6]

The lifeboats of the ship were of no help. Three of them had been lowered into the water, but they capsized because all the drowning men hung on to the sides in great clusters. A fourth boat still hung down the ship's side when the fire burned through the ropes. It crashed down and killed those swimming in the water.

An hour after the British attack, the *Cap Arcona* listed to port side, capsized, and pulled down with her into the depths a few hundred who had survived the fire. The wreck rose up on its starboard side, some twenty-five feet above the surface of the water. Over 300 men succeeded in pulling themselves back up to the hull, whose upper part was still burning hot. Only those who found a board could hang on there.

Now, finally, an hour and a half after the attack, the Standortkommandant of Neustadt, Frigate Captain Schmidt, sent two mine sweepers on rescue into Lübeck Bay. But the boats picked up only German soldiers and sailors. A Soviet prisoner, Aleksander Machnew, tried in vain to get into such a boat:

The Germans beat those who clung to the boat on their hands and mercilessly threw them back into the water. . . . The Germans started to shoot. With automatic weapons they shot at our comrades as they floundered in the water, and they sank silently in the depths.[7]

Still, there were some German sailors who showed themselves to be more humane. Paul Stassek, a photographer, writes:

I was able to persuade a young sailor at the railing to pull us on board, which was very hard to do. I was totally exhausted, and my right hand was injured. In order to escape further air attacks we sailed toward the naval experimental station at Pelzerhaken.[8]

Among those not taken on board the boat was the actor Erwin Geschonnek. He was able to swim back to the ship and pull himself up slowly on the anchor chain. That took an hour. Then he sat half frozen on the hull of the *Cap Arcona* together with the remaining 306 men. Icy rain started to fall. It was dusk. At around 7:00 p.m. the boats came. This time it was not the Germans, but the British, who in the interim had occupied Neustadt. They brought the survivors down from the hull, wrapped them in blankets, and took them ashore.

Though there were thirty or forty fishing boats in the harbor, not one of them had gone out to help the people on the sinking ships in the bay. And when that same evening those who had been rescued arrived in the city, most of its residents kept their doors shut. They ignored the knocking and pleading. Only a few dozen families took survivors into their homes and gave the starving and freezing concentration camp prisoners food and clothing. Even in Neustadt a little bit of human kindness existed here and there.

Six

If Kommandant Pauly had possessed that sense of responsibility of a Prussian officer he so often talked about, he should have been on the *Cap Arcona* and gone down with her. So said the deputy of the head of the Gestapo of Hamburg, SS-Sturmbannführer Rickert, in testimony before the British Military Tribunal.

> Defense Attorney Dr. König: "Were these people still under Pauly's command?"
> Rickert: "Yes."
> König: "So you regarded Pauly as the commanding officer of these people on the ship?"
> Rickert: "Yes."
> König: "And his responsibility for these people was not yet over?"
> Rickert: "Not as far as I know."
> König: "I want to make this perfectly clear. In your opinion these people were still under Pauly's command and he was responsible for getting them to their final destination?"
> Rickert: "He was charged with carrying out the orders of General Bassewitz-Behr, and he was therefore responsible for doing so."
> König: "Would it have been part of Pauly's duties to supervise the evacuation of such a large number of prisoners from Lübeck onto the ships? Would it have been a part of his duties?"
> Rickert: "I think that is quite self-evident."[1]

But Pauly had other things to do during those days. He was in charge of one of the last prisoners' kommandos that disposed of all traces of his crimes in Neuengamme. Almost half a ton of documents was burned, and a sign was put in front of the crematorium which read "Disinfection Room." The gallows were sawed off and thrown into the fire. The barracks were cleaned and whitewashed. They were

91

to make a good impression on the British. And that they did when on May 5, 1945, the first British soldier, a Lieutenant Charlton from Folkestone, walked through what had been Neuengamme concentration camp:

> We made a quick inspection of the prisoners' barracks and found them more or less clean and in order. There was no one there. It looked as if they had been cleaned in a hurry.[2]

Lagerkommandant Pauly then had some 2,000 parcels belonging to the Swedish Red Cross put on a truck. Jacobsen, the manager of the canteen, drove it to Westerdeichstrich (between Büsum and Wesselburen), to Pauly's home. There the truck stopped in front of a house on Ekenesch #2, where Pauly's parents-in-law lived. A portion of the 400,000 cigarettes, 20,000 bars of chocolate, and 20,000 packets of coffee and tea was unloaded. Pauly and Jacobsen (who ran an inn) divided the booty between themselves.

On May 3, Pauly drove his big olive-green service car first to Wesselburen and then on to Flensburg. There he went into hiding in the home of his sister-in-law, Anita Knuth, who lived on St. Jürgens Platz, on the corner of Ulmenstrasse. He threw away his Death's Head uniform and put on civilian clothing.

On May 15, 1945, at 11:00 p.m., the doorbell rang. Mrs. Knuth opened the door and two civilians asked if Max Pauly was there. They knew that he was. The men were from the British Army and were charged with searching out war criminals. They arrested Pauly and brought him to the internment camp at Neumünster.

The British also brought SS-Rottenführer Johann Frahm there, the man who had put the rope around the necks of the children in the boiler room of the school. He was hiding in his home village of Kleve, near Heide, in Holstein. Unterscharführer Willi Dreimann and Rottenführer Adolf Speck were apprehended in the area of Lübeck and also transported to Neumünster. Actually, these two, together with Unterscharführer Ewald Jauch, were to have brought the prisoners to the Baltic Sea. But instead Jauch had put on his civvies and run off into hiding to his home in Schwenningen, in the Black Forest. There he stayed hidden in his parents' home on Hauffstrasse #17 until the Military Police came, arrested him, and brought him to the British Internment Camp at Eselsheide, near Paderborn.

Three others still remained at large: Obersturmführer Arnold Strippel, SS-Doctor Kurt Heissmeyer, and Dr. Alfred Trzebinski.

Trzebinski was caught in February, 1946. He had packed an ambulance full with parcels belonging to the Swedish Red Cross and fled with them from Neuengamme. The murderer drove his big car past the flood of German troops returning from the misery of defeat, past the masses of bombed-out refugees and prisoners. He later complained in his diary that he had to jump into a ditch every time there was an air raid by the British, for

> there was no regard for the Red Cross and the Geneva Convention in this difficult phase of the war. We were able to spend a few more pleasant days with some farmers, where we had taken up lodgings; and when we left we gave them many fine things, such as a radio, a fur coat, etc.—things we did not want the enemy to have. And then we either had to surrender somewhere or go into hiding, because the British were all around us—the last bit of German soil had in the meantime become unfree.

That's the way he still saw it, even in his death cell—"unfree"—because the Allied Forces had come and taken power away from SS people like him.

Trzebinski found a hiding place with sympathizers in Husum. He writes:

> After much deliberation I decided to go underground in Husum, the "gray city" made famous by Theodor Storm's novellas. I was very well received and in a few days, with the gracious help of supporters, was able to exchange my SS uniform and insignia for those of the Wehrmacht and to work in the reserve military hospital as a Staff Physician of the Wehrmacht.

He was already starting to think that everything was forgotten. "Staff Physician" Trzebinski had himself transferred to an army hospital, and from there he went as an army doctor to the British discharging camp at Hesedorf, near Neumünster. He made this entry in his diary:

> Everything was just perfect. I was integrated into the German regular staff, and no one asked me for my papers. I received my military pay—my uniform with its borrowed insignia of the Wehrmacht gave me the necessary legitimacy. Not a soul in Hesedorf, neither British nor German soldier or civilian, had the faintest idea until the very end that in the innocent uniform of a

Staff Physician lay hidden a hunted, ostracized, outlawed SS
leader. In the adjoining room was the Intelligence Service, whose
task, among other things, was to apprehend people like me.
They, too, suspected nothing at all, and we were on the best of
terms. A Canadian First Lieutenant of this Intelligence Service
asked me to look for tattoos indicating blood types when examin-
ing persons to be dismissed. These were usually to be found
under the left arms of SS members, who could be identified
thereby even while wearing foreign uniforms. But in this instance
he unknowingly set a thief to catch a thief: I was blind to the blue
color of the tattoos. . . . My own blood type tattoo I had had
removed surgically by a colleague and friend in Husum. He, too,
must remain anonymous.

There are many such Trzebinskis who have similarly avoided
being caught. The doctor arranged for his wife and daughter to join
him, and they found rooms in Hesedorf's Hotel Wülpern. He hoped
to resume work as a doctor and no longer thought he would be
punished. What he did not know was that the British had established
a War Crimes Investigation Team in Bad Oeynhausen. There
Trzebinski's name appeared on the search list of a British major,
Anton Walter Freud. Freud spoke perfect German: The grandson of
Sigmund Freud, Anton Walter Freud had been born in Austria and
had emigrated to London. His maternal grandmother, who had
stayed behind in Vienna, was arrested there by the Nazis. She was
taken first to Theresienstadt and then to Auschwitz, where she was
gassed. She was well over eighty at the time.

Now her grandson had come back, too late to save her, but not
too late to confront the murderers: Höss, the Kommandant of Auschwitz, and Dr. Bruno Tesch, the industrialist from Hamburg who
had sold Cyclon-B to Auschwitz. "All of them unassuming, ordinary
people whom one could meet up with anywhere without having any
inkling of what they had done," Anton Walter Freud remembers
today.

Major Freud discovered that the trail of Dr. Trzebinski led to
Hesedorf. There the SS doctor was arrested on February 1, 1946, and
taken to the camp for war criminals at Westertimke. Trzebinski complains again in his diary:

To begin with, it was hammered into us to keep the prescribed
distance between us "Nazi pigs" and the culture-bearing soldiers

of the victorious armies: We had to stand at attention thirty paces before a British soldier approached us and thirty paces after he passed us by. That's more than was ever demanded in a German concentration camp.

Then the hearings began: What did he know of the fate of the twenty Jewish children? Nothing, Trzebinski insisted. But by this time Anton Walter Freud already knew that Trzebinski was there when the children where taken out of Neuengamme in a truck on April 20, 1945; the prisoners liberated from Neuengamme had told the British about the fate of the twenty children. Of course no one knew where they were, but as to who had taken them away, that the prisoners knew for certain: Dreimann, Trzebinski, Wiehagen, and Speck. And the prisoners demanded that the British interrogate these members of the SS about the fate of the children.

Speck was the first to admit knowing what happened to the children. On March 9, 1946, he declared the following under oath in the presence of H. P. Kinsleigh, a British captain, at the Neumünster camp:[3]

> Toward the end of April—I think it was the 20th—I was in my room around 8:00 p.m. I received an order from an SS man to come immediately to see Thumann in the protective custody camp. Unterscharführer Wiehagen, who was with me in my room, received the same order. We reported to the office of the Blockführer, and Thumann and Dreimann were there. Thumann ordered me to accompany to Hamburg a children's transport designated for the Swedish Red Cross.
>
> At about 8:30 p.m., the postal truck of Neuengamme pulled up in front of the sickbay. Perhaps twenty children between the ages of six and twelve were put inside. Two prison guards accompanied them. Another six adult inmates were also put in the truck. Wiehagen and I had to get in back. Dreimann and Trzebinski sat in front with the driver Petersen.
>
> We arrived at Bullenhuser Damm School at approximately 11:00 p.m. The adults got out first and went into the school with Dreimann and Trzebinski. Petersen, Wiehagen, and I stayed in the truck. Johann Frahm and Ewald Jauch were already there when we arrived. They both went into the school with Dreimann and Trzebinski and the six prisoners.

Trzebinski, Frahm, and Jauch then brought the twenty children into the school, together with the two prison guards.

About a half hour later—toward midnight—Trzebinski and, I believe, Dreimann came and ordered Wiehagen, Petersen, and me to get into the truck. We drove to the Spaldingstrasse auxiliary camp. Trzebinski got out and shortly thereafter twenty-five to thirty Russians were loaded into the truck. We then drove back to the Bullenhuser Damm School.

Wiehagen, Petersen, and I stayed in the truck. Trzebinski and Jauch brought four or six Russians into the school. A half hour later Trzebinski and Jauch came back out and brought four more Russians into the school. Again a half hour later Trzebinski and Jauch came back and wanted to bring in another four prisoners. Wiehagen stood to the left of the truck, I to the right, about five feet away.

The prisoners refused to come down off the truck. Trzebinski repeated his order. The prisoners tried to break loose. They all jumped off the truck at once and threw something in our eyes—I think it was salt. We were blinded for a moment and got into a scuffle. We made use of our weapons. I shot one Russian, Wiehagen shot two, and seven escaped. The rest were immediately taken into the school by Jauch and Trzebinski. Petersen stayed with the truck, and Wiehagen and I were ordered by Trzebinski to look for the others.

We looked for the seven escapees until four or five o'clock in the morning but returned without success. When we got back, Trzebinski was there by the truck. He ordered us to bring the bodies of the three who were shot down into the cellar. There we had to undress the bodies. The bodies of the other Russians were already lying there completely naked. I saw no signs of violence on them. I saw no bodies of the children in this cellar.

Petersen, Wiehagen, and I waited about half an hour for Trzebinski and Dreimann. About eight o'clock in the morning we drove back to Neuengamme. Jauch and Frahm stayed at the school.

On the same day, SS-Rottenführer Johann Frahm also testified before Captain Kinsleigh. Frahm was more precise and admitted to the murder of the children. But he put the principal blame on Trzebinski, whom the British had not yet found.

The children had to undress in a room down in the cellar. There Trzebinski gave each child, one after the other, an injection into the heart. Immediately thereafter each child was dead. The bodies were picked up the following day by truck.[4]

Anton Walter Freud, who now personally took over the interrogations, was a quiet and thorough worker. He questioned the imprisoned SS men over and over and confronted them with the statements of their fellow prisoners, thereby gradually obtaining more exact descriptions of the murder of the children. Frahm now declared that the Kommando had not gone directly to Bullenhuser Damm but first to Spaldingstrasse, to SS-Obersturmführer Strippel, who was to supervise the execution. He also admitted that Trzebinski did not kill the children by giving them injections into the heart but that he only drugged them with morphine injections, and that the children were then hanged.

Even after the trial against the principal defendants of Neuengamme had already begun, Anton Walter Freud continued to interrogate these SS men. On May 2, 1946, Johann Frahm spoke for the record and gave the most exact description of the children's murder:

> The Kommandoführer of Camp Bullenhuser Damm was Oberscharführer Jauch, and the Stützpunktleiter was Strippel. . . . I went down into the cellar where those newly arrived were gathered. There were approximately twenty children there between the ages of twelve and sixteen. Some of them seemed to be ill. Besides the children, Dr. Trzebinski, Dreimann, and Jauch were in the cellar. Strippel also came in every so often. The children had to undress in one of the rooms and were then taken to another room where they were injected by Dr. Trzebinski, so that they fell asleep. Those who still showed some signs of life after the injection were carried into another room. A rope was put around their necks and they were hung up on hooks like pictures on a wall. This was carried out by Jauch, me, Trzebinski, and Dreimann. Strippel was also present now and again. . . . At midnight another batch of prisoners arrived from Neuengamme. This time it was a group of twenty Russian men. They were taken into a room in the cellar and hanged by the four of us—Jauch, Trzebinski, Dreimann, and me, and in part also by Strippel. At six in the morning all the Russians were dead, and I went to sleep.[5]

Thus the prosecution was able to prove the murder of the children and convict the perpetrators.

The prosecutor was a British major, Stephen Malcolm Stewart. On March 18, 1946, the first legal proceedings were begun against the fourteen officials primarily responsible for Neuengamme concentration camp. Pauly was Defendant Number 1; Thumann, Number 3; Dreimann, Number 5; Speck, Number 9; and Trzebinski, Number 14. Four months later further legal action was initiated against Jauch and Frahm for child murder. At first, Strippel was also accused, but the proceedings against him were suspended. He had gone into hiding.

The British used as a courtroom one of the few halls that had not been destroyed in the bombed-out city of Hamburg—the hall in the Curiohaus, on the Rothenbaumchaussee. The proceedings thus became known as the Curiohaus trials.

In his prosecutor's address Major Stewart spoke about the official "Warning" that had been transmitted over the radio by the governments in London, Moscow, and New York on April 23, 1942. The message, directed to the "commanders, guards, and Gestapo officials in the German concentration camps," threatened them with severe punishment if they continued with their crimes. Then he went on to speak about the "Heissmeyer Children":

> Listen to the two witnesses who told the story of the French boy, Georges, and the French girl, Jacqueline, and the many other nameless children who were brought into the camp for these experiments. Listen to how they came into the camp completely healthy. They were lovely, normal, bright children. Then the experiments began. Small incisions were made in their arms and chests, and tubercle bacilli were rubbed in. In a few days the children became ill, and little Georges never left his bed again. Listen to how all these children were evacuated and murdered in Hamburg, together with the inmate doctor.

Major Stewart closed with these words:

> I know, Mr. President, that it is very difficult to contain one's human emotions when one hears about human beings who sank so low as to experiment with children and then to liquidate them. But I ask you, all the same, not to judge this charge in human

anger and indignation but only in accordance with the letter of the law.[6]

All the defendants tried to shift the guilt over the children's murder away from themselves.

Kommandant Max Pauly declared that he only carried out orders. After all, it was clear that every order had to be carried out, even an order that called for the execution of children.

However, that was not true. There were in Neuengamme not only people who obediently executed orders but also those who refused to do so. The prosecutor reminded Dr. Trzebinski of one such person, an inmate named Fritz Bringmann. He was an orderly. In February 1942, SS-Unterscharführer Willi Bahr had ordered him to kill Soviet prisoners of war by injecting them with phenol: "They're no longer able to work and have to be liquidated." Bringmann refused. "How was it possible for an inmate of a concentration camp to refuse the order of an SS man?" the prosecutor in the Curiohaus trial wondered. Bringmann, a Communist, answered him: "Because we political prisoners had character, and because it was an inhumane order."

In fact, he was not able to prevent the murder of the Russians. Bahr himself gave the fatal injections. Yet Fritz Bringmann had kept his humanity intact. He survived the concentration camp. He was never honored for his humane conduct.[7]

The SS understood something quite different by humaneness. Lagerkommandant Max Pauly, for instance, thought it was nothing more than caring for his own family. On May 3, 1945, he wrote a sentimental letter to his son, Hans-Werner, reminiscing about the time when his work in the concentration camp was financially rewarding:

> A beautiful house in Aldershorst,[8] completely free of debt—that's what your father could call his own. Besides that, your father was able to save some 25,000 marks at the Danzig and Rendsburg Savings Bank over a period of time. Add to that your own accounts. . . . How nice if I could be with all of you now.[9]

And Dr. Alfred Trzebinski complimented himself in notes he had made on May 24, 1946, in preparation for his testimony. Entitled "Events Regarding the Children's Murder," it reads:

I *cannot* reproach myself for giving the children a merciful injection of morphine before their execution. On the contrary, this was a humane act, of which I don't have to be ashamed.[10]

None of them was ashamed. They had all committed their crimes "for Germany," or "as soldiers." "Nothing is considered worthwhile today," Pauly writes to his son,

They say everything we did was bad. You can be as sure as a rock that I only did what I was ordered to do. It was a concentration camp authorized *by the state,* yet I am nevertheless held responsible for everything that higher-ups ordered me to do.[11]

Pauly wanted to put the responsibility for the children's murder on Dr. Trzebinski.

Defense Attorney Dr. Wessig: "Who issued the order?"
Pauly: "General Pohl."[12]
Wessig: "How did you learn of this order of execution?"
Pauly: "It was directed to the Standortarzt, and I read it at that time."
Wessig: "Did you receive this order of execution yourself and pass it on, or did the Standortarzt receive it directly?"
Pauly: "As I have already said, he received it directly. I don't remember if by letter or by teletype."
Defense Attorney Dr. Lappenberg: "And what did you tell Trzebinski on this occasion?"
Pauly: "I already said that I gave him the letter and told him to carry out the execution according to these orders."[13]
Lappenberg: "So he must have understood this as an order from you?"
Pauly: "He couldn't have, because I handed him the letter when it came."
Lappenberg: "What about the orderlies who took care of the children?"
Pauly: "They were included, because we considered all of them as one single unit."
Lappenberg: "You said that this was exclusively a matter for the medical department. Why then did the order come from General Pohl and not from the medical authorities?"
Pauly: "Possibly because Dr. Heissmeyer had conferred with

General Pohl on various occasions and because this station was
established as a medical station by order of General Pohl."

Lappenberg: "You deny that Dr. Trzebinski then refused to
carry out the order of execution of the children?"

Pauly: "Yes, I deny it."

Lappenberg: "Was there a discussion of how the children were to
be executed?"

Pauly: "As far as I remember, Trzebinski said it was his own
business."

Lappenberg: "Did Dr. Trzebinski tell you that he had no poison
for these injections?"

Pauly: "I can no longer remember that today."[14]

Chief Justice Stirling: "Could Trzebinski take along Dreimann
and Speck without your order?"

Pauly: "I assume they discussed that with the Lagerführer."

Stirling: "What happened to Professors Florence and Quenouille
who cared for the children?"

Pauly: "I don't know these two."

Stirling: "Are you sure you don't know them?"

Pauly: "Yes."

Stirling: "Did you realize that they were the most dangerous witnesses for what had been done to the children?"

Pauly: "It's possible."

Stirling: "Do you know if they were taken from Neuengamme or
not?"

Pauly: "Yes, they went with the children, because we also called
them medical attendants or orderlies."

Stirling: "When you speak of medical attendants or orderlies, do
you thereby include the two professors?"

Pauly: "Yes."

Stirling: "Then you admit that both of the professors left Neuengamme together with the children?"

Pauly: "As far as I know, four medical attendants went along;
whether or not two of them were professors, I don't know. At any
rate, four medical attendants went along with the children."

Stirling: "And what happened with the four medical attendants?"

Pauly: "They were executed."

Stirling: "How do you know that?"

Pauly: "That was included in the execution order."[15]

Pauly's inconsistent statements contradicted everything that the court had heard about executions in Neuengamme: orders for execution came from Berlin and were on principle directed to the Kommandant. He was the one who also had the responsibility for the murder of the children. During the actual carrying out of execution, the officer next in rank—the Lagerführer—had to be present. Normally this was SS-Obersturmführer Anton Thumann. But at noon on April 20, 1945, he had gone on to inspect the Wöbblin concentration camp in Mecklenburg. The officer next in rank after him was SS-Obersturmführer Arnold Strippel.

In his pleadings on behalf of Pauly, Pauly's attorney, Dr. Curt Wessig, who himself had been imprisoned by the Nazis in a protective custody camp, tried to clarify the role of the concentration camp commanders within the Nazi system. He called upon the court to recognize

> that Pauly had simply been a tool of a system that stormed through most of the countries of Europe in hate and fury, and that this system was bound to flounder because it refused to acknowledge and live out an ethics that called for the love of all that is human.

The court ought not to charge him with unproven accusations, Wessig continued. Nor does Pauly intend to admit "guilt for the fact that an autopsy was performed on a hanged Polish woman," Wessig explains in reference to the murder of the four attendants who had come from Auschwitz with the twenty children.

> Since the event has not been corroborated by any other witness, it cannot be considered proven, given defendant Pauly's statements to the contrary from the witness stand. Furthermore, whether the Polish women were executed according to law or whether or not a decision was rendered in their case by court-martial is a totally different question. It was, at any rate, against international law to execute a pregnant woman.[16]

According to Wessig, the murder of the children incriminated Pauly only insofar as he provided a transport truck; however, "Pauly had nothing to do with the atrocities that took place at Bullenhuser Damm." For this reason, Pauly stated he could not plead guilty in this matter as well.[17]

Prosecutor Major Stewart looked upon Pauly's guilt and that of his associates in a very different way:

> Pauly himself declared that he wanted to keep Heissmeyer at a distance, but without success. How can you reconcile this statement with a later one he made saying he knew nothing about the medical experiments on the adults? And then the experiments on the unfortunate children began. A singular kind of hypocrisy was used to deceive these children: they were given toys, and life was made easy for them, while at the same time they were being injected with tubercle bacilli. For four weeks these unfortunate, TB-infected children were observed in their prison by the staff—especially by the Kommandant, the Standortarzt, and the Lagerarzt. I cannot think of anything more despicable, more loathsome, than to experiment with unsuspecting children, and I don't think I have to say another word about the matter.

> Finally, as the Allies were approaching, a decision had to be made about the children. Pauly received the order and passed it on to Dr. Trzebinski by way of Thumann: the children should be executed. You will remember the conversation between Dr. Trzebinski and Pauly in which the Kommandant said to him: "Doctor, what do I hear? Are you too much of a coward to take charge of the children?" As if it took courage to murder twenty unsuspecting children.

> And finally, you have heard in all of its particulars one of the most terrible and gruesome testimonies of the whole trial, from witness Frahm and defendant Trzebinski. I don't want to repeat all the horrors in detail; but the children were brought to Bullenhuser Damm and, no matter how you want to look at it, no matter who it was who gave the order, no matter whose idea it was to poison them or to hang them, the fact still remains that they were murdered in cold blood in the cellar, in this very city. In my opinion, Dr. Trzebinski spoke the truth when he said, "You cannot execute children, you can only murder them." That is just what he did with the help of Frahm and the others.[18]

In conclusion, Chief Justice Stirling summed it up before retiring for deliberations:

> Pauly says that the order of execution was given directly to Dr.

Trzebinski, and Dr. Trzebinski says he never saw the order, that
it was given to the Kommandant. One must assume that an order
of this kind usually went to the Kommandant. . . . In any case,
Trzebinski told Strippel once again that he could not do it, but in
turn was told that he had to obey Pauly's orders. He says: "When
we arrived, Strippel, Jauch, and Frahm were waiting for us.
Strippel said everything was in order. . . ." Of all the dark and
brutal events in the history of the concentration camps the death
of the children in this cellar was one of the most brutal. If Dr.
Trzebinski, together with the others, is to be found guilty of the
death of the children, he must receive appropriate punishment.[19]

The court did not allow any of the defendants to claim innocence
on the basis of compulsory obedience to orders. On May 3, 1946, at
11:45 a.m., Chief Justice C. L. Stirling announced the verdicts: "Max
Pauly, the court sentences you to death by hanging." And the same
for Willi Dreimann, Adolf Speck, and Alfred Trzebinski—death by
hanging. Then the condemned men, who had been kept in Altona
prison until now, were transferred to the prison at Fuhlsbüttel, where
there were still death cells for those awaiting execution. They still had
another five months to live.

Max Pauly wrote the following to his son from his death cell:

My dear, dear boy, Always be proud of being a German, and
detest with all your might those who acquiesced in this absolutely
false verdict. . . . As for me, I find great consolation in the fact
that the German people as a whole unequivocally reject this per-
nicious propaganda of lies. . . . Please remember my favorite
dish—pancakes and chocolate pudding. If I could only eat my fill
once more! Keep your heads up high, dear ones! Your devoted
father.[20]

Dr. Alfred Trzebinski sought escape in his diary, entitled "I,"
where he took on the role of a good man. He describes an older
Danish woman who arrived at Neuengamme in April 1945, with the
white buses of the Danish Red Cross:

She stood at the camp gate, smoking a cigar. With her painted
lips she was blowing smoke rings nonchalantly into the faces of
the creatures who dragged themselves past her. Even in the concentration camp I never lost my delicate sense of tact. . . . Well, I

think that savages are at times far better than people who only pretend to possess tact.

The wife of Wilhelm Dreimann wrote this plea for clemency on behalf of her husband:

I cannot believe that my husband is to be punished for acts that were for him, after all, only orders. By this verdict you will make me and my child unhappy for the rest of our lives, and the punishment falls heaviest on us who are innocent. Both my child and I beg for leniency for my husband and the father of my child and ask you to rescind the death sentence.[21]

The Chief Justice of the British Army on the Rhine, Lord Bertrand Russell of Liverpool, rejected the plea for clemency. On August 26, 1946, the Commander-in-Chief of the British Army on the Rhine signed the eleven death sentences.

Five weeks later, on October 2, 1946, a British army truck pulled up to the Fuhlsbüttel prison. The condemned men had to get in. The unit drove from Hamburg to Hameln under heavy guard. There, in the prison, the executions were to take place.

Alfred Trzebinski wrote a letter of farewell to his wife:

Without having been an accomplice even once, I was dragged into things that were so totally foreign to my gentle nature that I not only rejected them outright but also tried with all my might to prevent them.

Despite my irreproachable, fair, and helpful attitude toward the former inmates, a caricature was made of me in the courtroom by criminal elements, who were incited and ready to commit perjury, as well as by common criminals, who had no scruples whatsoever. Although this did not, in fact, convince the court, it was nevertheless heard with pleasure. After all, the main purpose of this trial, in addition to convicting the other defendants, was to convict the Standortartz of Neuengamme as well, whether or not he was personally good or bad.

The court believed my statements almost to the word; but this was totally irrelevant to the court, because the Standortartz had already been found guilty even before the trial began—no matter if his name was Trzebinski or Schulze. . . . But if, after all possible attempts to save the children and after finally realizing that they could not be saved, not by anyone—if after all this I gave the children a merciful, weak injection of morphine, not to kill them but to ease their last hour before they were finally put to death by the hands of others, then this is a crime.[22]

On the morning of October 8, 1946, the prison chaplain led the first two of the condemned men into the death chamber. Present were the Chief Warden of the prison, Major Crapham, Captain Craig, and the British executioner, Albert Pierrepoint. At 10:59 a.m. the iron grate—on which the condemned men were standing with ropes around their necks—was released for the first time. During the next four hours two men were hanged every forty minutes. The last one died at 2:47 p.m.

Janssen, the prison chaplain, wrote to Willi Dreimann's widow, describing her husband's final hour:

It was very difficult for him to have to leave his loved ones. On his last night your husband took Holy Communion. I had the impression that he was very serious about this after all the waywardness of his life. For the sake of Jesus' death on the cross, may He have graciously accepted his plea: "God, have mercy on me, a sinner."

Dr. Trzebinski, even in the final moment of his life, felt that he was an innocent martyr, not a murderer of children. In his notebook Pierrepoint jotted down the last words of the doctor: "Lord, forgive them, for they know not what they do."

Two of the accused had escaped the hangman: Arnold Strippel and Dr. Kurt Heissmeyer.

Seven

Dr. Kurt Heissmeyer would probably never have been punished for his crimes against the children if a retired economist from Nuremberg had not bought a copy of *Stern* magazine on May 21, 1959. In its column "Dear STERN Reader," editor Jürgen von Kornatzky deplored the ignorance of German schoolchildren about the crimes of the Nazis:

> For example, one should tell the children in the classroom what happened some fourteen years ago in a Hamburg school that was used at the time as an auxiliary camp of Neuengamme concentration camp. Ten boys and ten girls from Jewish families, four to twelve years old, were kept in Neuengamme behind barbed wire and were used as a live breeding ground for SS-Dr. Heissmeyer's experiments with tubercle bacilli.

The economist knew the name Heissmeyer. In a letter to Hans Schwarz, the Secretary General of the Amicale Internationale de Neuengamme, he inquired if the Dr. Heissmeyer mentioned in *Stern* was "the same as lung specialist Dr. Kurt Heissmeyer who lived in Magdeburg, Gellertstrasse #12. As far as is known the latter was born 12/26/05; fled at some time to Magdeburg (not known from where); and married Eva H., born 1911, daughter of a minister."

Hans Schwarz forwarded this request to the Committee of Anti-Fascist Resistance Fighters in East Germany. There the identity of Heissmeyer was verified. Why another four years passed before Heissmeyer was arrested is not clear.

On the morning of December 13, 1963, officials of the East German General Prosecutor's Office rang the doorbell at Heissmeyer's home on Gellertstrasse #12. They produced an arrest warrant: suspicion of crimes against humanity. The doctor packed his things and was driven to a prison at Magdalenenstrasse #14 in Berlin for investigation.

Three days later Mrs. Eva-Renate Heissmeyer called on Dr. Wolfgang Vogel, an attorney in Berlin-Friedrichsfelde, and asked him to defend her husband. Vogel thus made the acquaintance of one of those successful provincial doctors who quickly attained middle-class prosperity and prestige at a time when there were very few physicians in East Germany. Heissmeyer had a large practice and the only private TB clinic in the country. He owned a nice house filled with expensive furniture, antiques, paintings, and carpets. The son of a country doctor and a pastor's daughter had established a thriving family. Their three children were well provided for: their father had bought his two sons and one daughter each a house.

Dr. Kurt Heissmeyer, who had turned fifty-nine the day after Christmas that year, was considered a good doctor in Magdeburg. He was always accessible to his patients, and people initially suspected that he had been arrested simply because of his political views. It was known that he stood on the right—raised in a reactionary home in Sandershausen, Thuringia; all members of his family had been more or less sympathetic to fascism; his uncle had even been an SS general and had been married to the head of the Women's League of the Reich, Gertrud Scholz-Klink. While a student in Marburg, Heissmeyer had joined a duelling fraternity called "Arminia" and later wrote about it in a biographical statement:

> I was convinced that conditions in the Weimar Republic were intolerable. Consequently, I felt myself all the more committed to the goals of the fraternity, which found their expression in such slogans as "God—Freedom—Fatherland" and in words expressive of discipline and honor.

An anti-Semite, an early member of Hitler's party, and later an officer in the SS—not exactly a model citizen of a state of workers and farmers. Nevertheless, could Kurt Heissmeyer really be a criminal?

At first Heissmeyer denied everything that he was accused of. Criminal experiments on human beings? True, he acknowledged he had carried out experiments but strictly in accordance with medical ethics. In fact, he could provide proof even now, he said, for in April 1945 he had buried a box in the garden of his house in Hohenlychen containing the documentation of his experiments. This box would surely still be intact today, nineteen years after the end of the war, because it was lined with zinc.

Prosecutors Nienkirchen and Friedrich drove to Hohenlychen with a pioneer group of the People's Army. Heissmeyer showed them the spot where the box was buried. The mine detector belonging to the pioneers indicated buried metal.

Heissmeyer had not lied. The box was dug up. Inside were pieces of silverware and a photograph album entitled "Our Child," with pictures of his oldest son. They also found an outline of a scientific paper, cans containing 35 mm films, X-ray photographs, temperature graphs, and a porcelain dish of limited edition bearing an inscription from Hebbel's poem "Die Weihe der Nacht." On the reverse side it read: "1944. To you and your clan. I wish you a Blessed Yuletide and a Happy New Year. Pohl, SS-Obergruppenführer and General der Waffen-SS." (This was the same "Blessed Yuletide" during which the inmates of Neuengamme made wooden toys for the "Heissmeyer Children" and gave them caramel candies to ease their misery.)

The X-ray photographs were submitted to Dr. Schubert, a senior physician at the Berlin Charité, for his evaluation. He found changes in three photos that were probably caused by an "inoculation into the lungs":

> Case Number 10066 Morgenstern, Jacqueline (probe?). There is apparently no change in the right lung. On the left the diaphragm is obscured by density in the lateral lung fields. This density extends from the diaphragm to the anterior fourth rib. . . . One cannot exclude the possibility that this condition developed because of an "inoculation" of tubercle bacilli into the left lung.

A similar finding was made in the case of Lelka Birnbaum ("dense shadow in the lower right lobe, as appears in adults when given an inoculation of tubercle bacilli into the lungs . . ."), and also in the case of Sergio de Simone (". . . the condition could well have been caused by an 'injection into the lungs' . . .").

This was not information that would exonerate Heissmeyer, who had endangered his own life by mentioning the box, since such experiments were crimes against humanity, still punishable in East Germany by death. Heissmeyer's attorney, Dr. Wolfgang Vogel, knew from his own experience that such punishment was no empty threat:

his former client, concentration camp physician Dr. Horst Fischer, had been sentenced to death and executed in East Germany for carrying out selections among inmates in the India rubber factory of IG Farben at Auschwitz-Monowitz concentration camp.

Heissmeyer no longer tried to deny his crimes. In a hearing on March 10, 1964, he admitted that he had looked upon people as guinea pigs.

> Prosecutor Nienkirchen: "Why did you conduct your experiments in a concentration camp?"
> Heissmeyer: "It was clear to me that the use on human beings of the serum available to me was really not justifiable owing to the possible consequences. I thought I could justify it in the concentration camp because I looked upon the inmates of the camp as second-class citizens, given my strong affirmation of Nazism at the time. I knew that the inmates and the children in the camp were at the mercy of the SS, and so I did not have to ask them first if they would put themselves at my disposal for medical testing. Had the experiments produced negative results, there would have been no legal consequences for me. Furthermore, these experiments were conducted in a concentration camp because such experiments, utilizing people instead of animals, were not intended to be made public.[1]

At another hearing Heissmeyer elaborated:

> As a physician I knew, of course, that I really was not permitted to do this, and outside of a concentration camp it hardly would have been possible. At the same time, the lives of these people would be endangered. So as not to have these possible consequences be made public, I conducted my experiments in a concentration camp. At any rate, my attitude in those days was such that I did not think inmates of a camp had full value as human beings.

Did he think his human subjects might die? Heissmeyer:

> The inmates of the Neuengamme concentration camp, as well as the children brought there in the fall of 1944 at my request, were simply experimental objects for me. I would also like to state that the inmates on whom I experimented died more quickly than might otherwise have been the case.

On April 6, 1964, Heissmeyer was interrogated specifically about the experiments on children. Heissmeyer:

Today I realize that by conducting experiments on the children I committed—I'd like to say—a crime against humanity, because these children were totally defenseless, and my experiments should actually have required the consent of the guardians. But at that time I did not give this any thought; because of my fascistic convictions I regarded neither the inmates of the concentration camp nor the children as complete human beings.

In January 1965, the hearings were in essence concluded. The prosecutor asked Dr. Heissmeyer if he wanted to give his own assessment of his human experiments. On January 19, 1965, the doctor formulated a series of "Comments on Medical Experiments I Conducted in Neuengamme Concentration Camp." Reading them, one gets the idea that these terrible experiments had somehow served the good of humanity:

I was convinced at that time that all those who were sentenced to death would not escape their fate, regardless of whether the experiments were carried out or not. Now I believe that I would have been allowed to conduct these experiments, such as they were, even then at a public institution without making myself liable for punishment. I have always been conscious of the fact that I gained valuable knowledge in Neuengamme that helped my future patients and, indeed, was a blessing for them many times over.

Last but not least I learned to observe psychological processes at Neuengamme, as paradoxical as that may seem. And if I have become a good doctor at all, my strengths may be found in my recognition of such processes, and some part of that I also have Neuengamme to thank for. What I learned there, other colleagues of mine in private practice often had to acquire in difficult circumstances and without the possibility for clinical observation—in the beginning not always such a good thing for the patients.

Thus Heissmeyer faulted his colleagues for their relative inexperience because they themselves had not conducted human experiments in concentration camps. After the fact he wanted to give "meaning" to his crime.

After two and a half years of investigatory detention, Dr. Kurt Heissmeyer was brought to trial on June 21, 1966, before the court in Magdeburg. The indictment was not murder but "crimes against humanity." In East Germany, in contrast to West Germany, the London Statute for the International Military Tribunal of August 8, 1945, is the law in force. This statute created the legal basis, after the end of the Nazi regime, for the "just and expeditious trial and punishment of major war criminals." Since then nineteen member nations of the United Nations have joined in this agreement, but not West Germany. In Article 6, Paragraph c of the statute, "crimes against humanity, namely murder, extermination, enslavement, deportation, or other inhuman acts" are liable for punishment.

Heissmeyer described to the court how he came to join the SS: 1933—training, first in Freiburg, then in the famous Swiss Mountain clinic of Davos-Clavadel; resident in Auguste-Victoria Hospital in Berlin; after 1938 Senior Physician in the TB Sanatorium of Hohenlychen (in the Uckermark), which was later taken over by the SS.

"I asked myself how anybody could keep on being just a Senior Physician," Heissmeyer's colleague, Professor Hans Klein, who had been head of pathology at Hohenlychen, recalls today.

> He was already older than I, and a ponderous person. His face showed little expression. He was unable to articulate his thoughts; Professor Gebhardt never invited Heissmeyer to anything, not even official gatherings. He just tagged along. The only patron Heissmeyer had was his uncle, August, the SS-Obergruppenführer. Gebhardt never liked Heissmeyer and only tolerated him because he had to. Heissmeyer suffered because of this; he always wanted to be something more. He was always under pressure. The others all succeeded, only he did not.

The scholarly standing of a physician was and continues to be measured by the number and quality of his publications. Except for two short papers displaying the ignorance of a layman, Heissmeyer produced nothing. In order to become a somebody, he had to do what "all the others" around him were doing, namely conduct human experiments. The "material"—defenseless victims—was available to him and his colleagues in the nearby concentration camps of Ravensbrück and Sachsenhausen. For example, Heissmeyer's superior, Professor Karl Gebhardt,[2] conducted experiments that sought a cure for gas gangrene, which occurs following gunshot wounds. For that the doctors had their patients shot at, in order to simulate "the conditions existing on the front," in the words of Gebhardt's Senior Physician, Dr. Fritz Fischer. Heissmeyer's colleague, Dr. Hertha Oberheuser, worked on a cure for artificially induced bone fractures. Women placed on an operating table had both of their lower thighs broken with a hammer. And Dr. Stumpfegger's specialty was the transplanting of bone from inmates to wounded SS personnel. Once an entire shoulderblade was transplanted on a wounded man named Franz Ladisch. After their bones were thus removed, inmates were immediately put to death by injection.

Dr. Heissmeyer also was required to do "scientific" work, for without presenting such work about his own experiments, he could become neither an Instructor nor a Professor of Medicine. His goal was to disprove the theory held by Robert Koch and Rudolf Virchow that tuberculosis was purely an infectious disease. Kurt Heissmeyer maintained that only an "exhausted" organism was receptive to such infection, most of all the "racially inferior" organism of the Jews. Thus the need for Jewish subjects for his experiments.

He did not have any moral inhibitions against such human experiments, for according to the "philosophical theory of folk and race, it is not feasible to deduce the origin of human tuberculosis from experiments on animals, for such a procedure suggests that the constitution of animals is the same as that of man." This is what he wrote in 1943 in an essay that was considered to be "so primitive in its overall conception that it could well have been written by a layman of limited ability," in the judgment of Otto Prokop, Professor of Forensic Medicine.

In the Magdeburg trial the medical ignorance of the defendant became especially apparent. Prokop asked him: "Where did you obtain your knowledge of immunology?" Heissmeyer could not give an answer. Prokop asked: "Who were your instructors in microbiology and immunology?" Heissmeyer could not come up with any names. Prokop asked: "What scientific textbooks on bacteriology have you read?" Heissmeyer knew of none. Prokop: "Just give me any title." Heissmeyer could not remember any.

Prokop: "Why did you conduct these experiments?"
Heissmeyer: "Because one had to find out if there was any immunization against TB."
Prokop: "If you were of the opinion that Jews were more dis-

posed to TB than Aryans, why then did you experiment with Jews at all? According to your theory it's not even possible to apply the results to Aryans. Why didn't you use guinea pigs?"
Heissmeyer: "For me there was no basic difference between human beings and guinea pigs."
Then he corrected himself: "Between Jews and guinea pigs."

As precedent he recalled that two Austrian TB researchers—H. and A. Kutschera-Aichbergen, father and son—had conducted similar TB experiments between 1929 and 1941. But these experiments had not produced results and were, in fact, considered obsolete at the time Heissmeyer began his own. The Austrians, moreover, had never experimented on healthy subjects and certainly not on children. And nothing could ever justify the torturous and life-threatening inoculation of live bacterial strains into the lungs. "There is no basis whatsoever for assuming that the introduction of virulent tubercle bacilli into the lungs could have any sort of usefulness," A. Kutschera-Aichbergen wrote, appalled when he heard that Heissmeyer had invoked his authority.[3]

Heissmeyer himself had to admit that what he was doing was worthless. At the latest, he realized the senselessness of his work in October 1944, when the experiments with the adult inmates were completed. Nonetheless, he had the children sent on from Auschwitz and exposed them to a death that he himself felt was senseless. He declared for the record:

> After determining in the fall of 1944 that my plan to heal TB patients with the above-mentioned serum had failed, and that the condition of most of the inmates had worsened and not improved, I discontinued the experiments. I then ordered twenty children to be brought in on whom I used the same serum to see if they were inherently immune to TB as well as to see if I could immunize them against the disease.

Only after the war, he said, did he learn that the children were actually murdered:

> These experiments continued until April 1945, at which time the children were taken away from me and murdered by the SS, as I learned after the war from the book Geissel der Menschheit.[4]

Otto Prokop, an expert in forensic medicine, worked for four months to prepare his report on "The Human Experiments of Kurt

Heissmeyer, M.D."[5] "It was a key experience for me. For the first time
the crimes of the Nazis became clear to me," he later recounted.

> I have not seen anything worse in my practice of forensic
> medicine. When my secretary was taking down the account of the
> children and their deaths she cried, and that's something when
> you consider that she was used to taking notes during autopsies.[6]

Prokop knew very well that his professional opinion had political
implications. Many physicians were still skeptical of the East German
government at that time. They were not sure if Heissmeyer had really
committed a crime or if he had been brought to trial because of his
reactionary past. The Magdeburg Medical Association had sent ob-
servers to the courtroom, but Prokop addressed a challenge to the
entire body of his colleagues. After the sentencing he gave a lecture
about Heissmeyer's experiments to a packed house in the Hotel International in Magdeburg:

> His desire to undertake experiments on people with TB patho-
> gens contradicted all the basic concerns and ethical duties of a
> physician, even according to existing regulations and official
> views in force at the time. A circular prepared by the
> Reichsminister of the Interior dated February 18, 1931 . . . states
> in principle that every new medical treatment must be in accor-
> dance with the principles of medical ethics and that representa-
> tives of medicine and science must conform to these
> principles. . . . Experiments on children or on the young are not
> permitted if these endanger them even in the least.

Prokop then quoted from the professional opinion that he had presented to the court:

> One characteristic feature of Heissmeyer's experiments is his
> extraordinary lack of concern; add to this his gross and total
> ignorance in the field of immunology, in particular bacteriology.
> He did not then, nor does he now, possess the necessary expertise
> demanded of a specialist in TB diseases. The defendant showed
> no knowledge of Mendel-Mantoux, as was evident at the trial.
> The name meant nothing to him. He knew nothing about the
> serum developed by Boehma; nor could he name a single text-
> book on bacteriology that he could have based his investigations
> on at the time. And he does not know any modern bacteriology
> textbook. He was also not familiar with work methods in bac-

teriology. Neither he nor his medical assistant Kirst[7] wore protective masks when preparing the suspensions of bacteria. Some of the cultures that were used stood around freely in the laboratory. . . . Conditions in the barracks where the experiments were going on were most conducive to infection. From time to time attempts were made to disinfect the premises, but the materials used were insufficient against TB. . . . One cannot detect in these experiments any of the medical care and scrupulous attitude expected of doctors. . . . Professor Steinbrück, Dr. Schubert, and Dr. Landmann have presented extensive data from the medical records that show that these experiments were useless for scientific research and that they in no way enriched it. . . . According to his own admission Heissmeyer was not concerned about curing the prisoners who were put at his disposal. Nor did he believe that his experiments would produce therapeutic results, and he actually counted on their being detrimental, indeed even fatal, to the prisoners. Given conditions in the concentration camps, Heissmeyer was not afraid that he would have to account for the consequences of his actions, for his own personal interests were in full accord with those of the fascist rulers.[8]

But Heissmeyer was suspected of something far worse still: Had he perhaps urged the SS leadership in Berlin to murder the children and thus remove the traces of his crimes? Kommandant Pauly had voiced this suspicion at the Curiohaus trial.

Heissmeyer denied this. He had nothing to do with the murders, he said, but was fleeing from Hohenlychen on April 21, 1945, as the Red Army was approaching. He was wearing civilian clothing and going under an assumed name. Later he returned to Sangershausen, in Thuringia, where for a time he helped his father, a country doctor, in his medical practice.

Then Dr. Kurt Heissmeyer went to Magdeburg under his own name and opened a practice on Gellertstrasse #12 as a lung specialist. He began a new life.

It was a new life indeed. Dr. Kurt Heissmeyer the lung specialist of Magdeburg seemed to have nothing in common with Heissmeyer the SS-doctor.

Defense Attorney Vogel: "It cannot be disputed that for about twenty years the defendant did the opposite of what he now stands accused of."

A dozen patients declared in court that Heissmeyer had cured them and saved their lives. Erich Albrecht, a witness from Magdeburg: "Because of Dr. Heissmeyer's conscientious treatment I am still able to work, despite my sixty-eight years, in a managerial capacity at a people's plant." Another witness, Siegfried Schubert: "Dr. Heissmeyer was able to save my life because he immediately initiated treatment that lasted seven years." Margarete Nieke, a witness from Magdeburg: "I had a huge cavity in my lung and had lost all hope when I turned to Dr. Heissmeyer for help. And I found it, too." Witness Lisbeth Paul: "I have Dr. Heissmeyer to thank for being alive today; if it were not for him, I would have died long ago. He was like a father to those of us who were ill." Erna Heiges: "Dr. Heissmeyer was ready day and night to help his patients. Thanks to him I am back at work once again."

There were two persons on trial in the Magdeburg court: a self-sacrificing doctor under one kind of regime, and a criminal without regard for human life under another. He was like thousands of those who did not resist a criminal system. He lacked all standards of humaneness. Dictatorship can count on people like Kurt Heissmeyer.

"He does not stand here before the court as a participant in the fascist program of annihilation," his defense attorney, Dr. Wolfgang Vogel, pleaded.

> He was not a hangman in a white coat, not Standortarzt. It was not his concern to participate in the Final Solution of the Jewish Question. He was only concerned with having free rein in his pseudo-scientific obsession, which had so ruined his medical ethos that he didn't think twice about equating people with rabbits. This obsession, though he may not admit it, can be explained by his determined quest for academic honors.

This quest for recognition was typical of a certain large segment of the German middle class, the defense counsel asserted.

> The defendant had been shaped not only as a human being but also as a physician by his nationalistic and later pro-fascist environment. He was raised as a nationalist. It was drummed into him that the German people were not yet ripe for becoming a republic. In 1937 he joined the NSDAP. He published an article on folk and race. And today he says this about himself: "I saw in Hitler a strong personality, a man right for the times. I found the

racial policies against the Jews to be correct. The war against
Russia seemed to me a continuation of the battle with other
weapons. Above all, in Hohenlychen I felt I had become more
and more nationalistic. Starting with Hitler and going on to
Himmler, Hess, and so on—the whole bunch of Nazis in Hohenlychen were all in it together." A concentration camp was situated
about seven miles down the road: this "brown-shirt" mind-set
could not remain without influence on the thinking and behavior
of the defendant. The atmosphere at Hohenlychen was aptly
described for posterity by Dr. Gebhardt in his favorite saying:
"The man of character goes his own way; he who has none remains my servant." Allow us, then, to make the following statement: Heissmeyer was a product of his time, even as a doctor in
his white coat.

Thus, Dr. Wolfgang Vogel did not present the picture of a born
criminal, of a Satan, but of a gentle burgher from the German middle
class who is loyal to the state unto its very last crime. This should not
be forgotten in West Germany, which no longer considers a person's
anti-Semitic youth and early participation in the NSDAP a hindrance
for even the highest of public offices.

In summing up, Dr. Vogel stated that Heissmeyer's guilt for the
death of the children had not been proven, because

> to hold the defendant criminally responsible it is not enough to
> argue that the experiments on the children provide an objective
> cause for murder. Causality in criminal law is not to be con-
> sidered as being merely objective. Both the objective and the
> subjective facts of a statutory offense need to be considered for a
> decision to be reached. And such accord is lacking in the evidence
> given by the witnesses, in the case of the murdered Jewish chil-
> dren as well.

On the other hand, Dr. Vogel did admit that in three cases Heissmeyer's experiments on the adults was the cause of death:

> In view of the evidence, in view of the opinion of the experts, in
> view of the testimony of the witnesses, but also in view of the
> contestation offered by the defendant, we are unable to invali-
> date the claims of the prosecutors. However, it is our duty to

point out that these three instances of death do not qualify as murder according to the norms of the criminal code.

And for that reason Defense Attorney Dr. Vogel petitioned that Heissmeyer not be given a death sentence, nor life imprisonment, but only a jail term.

What Heissmeyer had to say in his closing words had already been recorded in his final statement:

> The fact remains—healthy people were made ill. I am aware of that. If, then, twenty years later, I am nevertheless unable to feel remorse—and this is probably what is asked and expected of me—then it is because twenty years have passed, and in those twenty years I have not been inactive. Moreover, I expect that if one is to judge fairly, one should weigh the bad deeds against the good, and this might perhaps prove that I helped more patients than I did not. Add to this my conviction that I did not intend anything bad with these experiments and did not commit anything bad, if one disregards the concentration camp.

On June 30, 1966, after six days of trial proceedings, the court passed judgment: Dr. Kurt Heissmeyer was sentenced to life imprisonment in a penitentiary. "By operating on the children the defendant showed no human emotions whatsoever, since he himself admitted that given his fascist orientation he saw no difference between a guinea pig and a Jewish child."

Dr. Kurt Heissmeyer was sixty years old at the time. He was put in prison at Bautzen. His attorney, Dr. Vogel, remembers: "About a year after the sentencing Frau Eva Heissmeyer came to me and asked me to submit a plea for clemency for her husband because he had heart trouble. Then came the news of his death." On August 29, 1967, Kurt Heissmeyer died of a heart attack.

His two sons also became doctors. They had grown up with their sister and a young boy with TB, whom Heissmeyer had taken in as a foster child. One of his sons says of his father's deeds: "I am still grappling with all of this: How can a man who loved children so much do such a thing?"

Eight

In January 1964, Dr. Helmut Münzberg, Chief Prosecutor of Hamburg, received a letter from Rudolph Gottschalk, the chairman of the Arbeitsgemeinschaft Buchenwald in Frankfurt:

> We would like to know if an inquiry has been made or an indictment served on former SS-Hauptsturmführer Strippel[1] because of his decisive role in the murder of the children at the Hamburg school of Bullenhuser Damm; and if so, with what results.

Accompanying the letter was a pamphlet entitled "The Bell of Ettersberg. Journal of Former Inmates of the Buchenwald Concentration Camp on the Ettersberg, near Weimar."

In this journal, under the headline "The Elite of the German Nation," a report appeared about SS-Führer Strippel and his participation in the murder of the children at Bullenhuser Damm:

> The children's murderers, as many as could be apprehended, were hanged. But in none of the Neuengamme trials, nor in the so-called Drütte trial held before the British Military Tribunal in Lüneburg, was SS-Hauptsturmführer Strippel, head of the SS special units of Spaldingstrasse and Bullenhuser Damm, ever prosecuted. He had disappeared without a trace in the chaos that accompanied Germany's collapse.

Prosecutor Münzberg, thirty years old at the time, did not know the name Strippel. Although Münzberg was born in Hamburg, had gone to school there, and had worked in the special office for Nazi crimes, he had never heard anything about the murder of children at Bullenhuser Damm. He could not find any documents on this crime in the prosecutor's office or in the state archives. It was as if there had never been a Curiohaus trial by the British military authorities. There

120

were no documents on Neuengamme concentration camp. Fifty-five thousand people had been murdered there, but the Hamburg judiciary had not taken notice of the biggest crime in the history of the city.

This was the case not only in Hamburg.[2] The German Parliament discussed granting a "general amnesty for all crimes committed during the Hitler era."[3]

A member of Parliament and later Minister of Justice, Joachim von Merkatz, as early as 1952 had demanded of the government through Parliament that "a solution to the question of the so-called 'war criminals' should be a prerequisite for facilitating Germany's consent to contribute to defense." (The phrase "so-called" before "war criminals" makes it seem as if it had been simply a matter of war crimes to gas millions of Jews or to hang twenty children.)

Konrad Adenauer had been the first to say that the rearming of West Germany would only be possible once the criminals of the last war were no longer put on trial. In August 1950, in an official memorandum, Adenauer had his representative, ex-Wehrmacht General Hans Speidel, declare that "the pardoning of the war criminals and the termination of the defaming of German soldiers" has to be "the prerequisite for our every military contribution."[4]

Then he sent Generals Speidel and Heusinger to a secret meeting, at night, at the residence of the American High Commissioner, McCloy, the representative of the occupying powers. "Only when they had taken off their heavy winter coats did I recognize the men as Heusinger and Speidel, "American diplomat Charles W. Thayer said.[5] "They somberly confirmed that if the Landsberger defendants were to be hanged, the German defense pact against the East would remain nothing more than a hope."

The defendants who were sentenced to death in the Nuremberg trials were waiting at that time on death row in the prison at Landsberg, on the Lech River. That is where the executions by hanging also took place.

The reaction of the Americans to the pressure exerted by Adenauer came quickly. Even though a few of those convicted were executed, such as SS-General Pohl in June 1951, for example, amnesties and pleas for clemency soon followed. "A rash of pleas for clemency broke out," wrote Robert Kempner, the former American prosecutor in the Nuremberg trials. Most of those condemned were quietly set free. Of the thirteen who were condemned to death, all former members of the Einsatzgruppe Ohlendorf—a mobile death squad that had destroyed many hundreds of thousands of Jews in Poland—only four were hanged. The other nine were able to return home free after only a few years' imprisonment.[6]

Then the German courts were given jurisdiction for handling concentration camp crimes, and from then on silence reigned about the mass murders. With the vigorous approval of the German Bundestag, Social Democratic Party representative Merten declared on September 17, 1952: "We must stop all discrimination against Germans, including that before the law. We must stop the application of justice based on the desire for revenge and dictated by retribution."

Silence reigned because one of those responsible for the extermination of the Jews, Dr. Hans Globke, had been appointed by Adenauer to the highest office in the Federal Republic. He had been an official in charge of Jewish Affairs in Hitler's Ministry of the Interior. He had ordered the stamping of Jewish passports with a "J," the compulsory introduction of the first names of "Sarah" and "Israel," the wearing of the Jewish Star, and various measures for the resettlement of the Jews.[7]

This man was now Secretary of State of West Germany, responsible for drawing up the agenda for cabinet meetings, drafting the bills of the ministers, and influencing public opinion. Besides the Secret Service, he also controlled the "Reptilienfonds," secret government funds not subject to public control. He used this fund to bribe journalists and newspapers, such as the radical right-wing *Deutsche Soldatenzeitung*, which received 11,000 marks per month.[8]

In February 1961, there was indeed a pretrial investigation of Globke, for he was suspected of having prevented 10,000 Jewish women and children from leaving Greece for Israel and of having handed them over instead to Eichmann, and to their destruction. However, the prosecutor's office in Bonn quickly stayed the investigation. On the other hand, Globke was accused in 1963 before the East German Supreme Court in Berlin of having been involved in the murder of millions of Jews. Four thousand documents were read, and Globke was sentenced in absentia to life imprisonment. However, speaking for the Federal Government in Bonn, then Secretary of State von Hase (today director of a German television broadcasting corporation) declared that the show-trial that recently opened in East Berlin against Secretary of State Dr. Globke exclusively serves the aims of Communist propaganda directed against the Federal Republic. It is obviously intended to be the climax of what has been for years a systematic harassment of the closest aides of the Chancellor. The charges have proven to be totally unfounded.

They were certainly not all that unfounded, however, for even conservative Switzerland prohibited Globke from ever entering that country, when he wanted to move into his Swiss villa upon retirement.

The West German bureaucracy resisted the concentration camp trials. This stand was expressed most clearly by the country's chief prosecutor after he stepped down from office, former Federal Attorney General Max Güde. As a member of the Christian Democratic Party he criticized two prosecutors who traveled to Moscow to examine murder records: "Our idiots even go *there* and bring back that stuff!"[9]

In the meantime, the criminals themselves had slipped under the shield of a protecting bureaucracy—the police, the judiciary, the administration, and the army. On September 1, 1956, on the seventeenth anniversary of Hitler's invasion of Poland, the Defense Minister in Bonn announced a "general dispensation"[10] that enabled former members of the Waffen-SS up to the rank of SS-Obersturmbannführer to join the West German Army. That was the rank held by most of the concentration camp commanders at the end of the war, including Max Pauly.

In light of these circumstances, then, it is no wonder that Chief Prosecutor Münzberg of Hamburg could find no documents about the murder of the children at Bullenhuser Damm: "I had a great deal of difficulty before I finally located the minutes of the Curiohaus trial in the cellar of the British Embassy in Bad Godesberg." These were by no means complete, as became evident many years later. But Münzberg also found Arnold Strippel: he was serving time in Butzbach prison, with a soft job in the prison infirmary. In finding Strippel, Münzberg uncovered as well the life story of a German concentration camp guard.

"I, Arnold Strippel, was born on June 2, 1911, in Unshausen, in the district of Kassel. I was the second son of a farmer, Friedrich

Strippel, and his wife Martha, née Wald," he writes in his autobiographical statement for the SS Race and Resettlement Department.[11]

> From age six to fourteen I attended the elementary school there. After leaving school I learned the carpenter's trade in my uncle's building business. Three years later, even though I had passed my apprenticeship examination, I stayed on with my master, and later, when the building trade was in a depression, I went to work on my parents' farm. In the spring of 1934, I applied for admission to the regular SS. On June 1, 1934, I was inducted into the SS-Sonderkommando "Sachsen," which later was integrated into what became the Death's Head Units.

Like most of the concentration camp guards then, Strippel came out of the reserve army of the jobless—as did Dreimann, Speck, Jauch, and even Pauly. Arnold Strippel was accepted by the SS. Inside and out, he met the requirements of this Blood Order: dark blond, Germanic looking, and six feet tall, someone whom Dr. Blies, a concentration camp physician, described as "stately in posture," "Nordic" in appearance, with "rosy-white" skin. He is described in similar terms by numerous prisoners of his in the German concentration camps. And there are only a few such camps that Strippel did not set foot in in the course of his career.

He started out in October 1934 as one of the guard troops of the Sachsenburg concentration camp in Saxony. In 1938 he was already Rapportführer in Buchenwald concentration camp, near Weimar. Among his duties was the punishment of prisoners. "Flogging was administered on the sawhorse, over which the prisoner was placed with his back strapped down," as was established in 1949 at the Frankfurt murder trial, when the court announced its verdict against Strippel. "The punishment consisted of five to twenty-five blows. In the beginning, canes the thickness of a finger were used; from the end of 1930 on, short leather whips; and finally, bull whips."

Even more effective was something called "tree-hanging."

> The prisoners were hung on a tree—their backs against the bark, their arms tied together—a posture which produced extreme pain and usually pulled their arms out of their sockets. The victims had to hang many hours in this torturous position and afterwards were not able to use their arms for months and had to be fed by their fellow inmates.[12]

The verdict continues:

The defendant himself has admitted that as Rapportführer he announced to the inmates such punishments as beatings on the sawhorse and tree-hangings, and that he was present when these punishments were meted out. According to his declarations, these functions were part of his duties. But beyond that it has been determined that the defendant himself physically took part in the administering of these punishments, and on other occasions mistreated the inmates at will. . . . He even let it happen that prisoners now and then remained tied and hanging from the tree throughout the night, and he permitted them to be taken down from this painful position only the next morning, according to witness Zannwetzer. . . . Strippel was considered a brutal type of mercenary and was feared by everyone in the camp. He was known among the inmates as a man who did not hesitate to act, and he showed himself at his worst in committing atrocities. He gained inner satisfaction from bullying and torturing the concentration camp inmates whenever he could.

Witness Zannwetzer continued to say in a firm and convincing manner: "Strippel was a man who considered it of the highest importance to do his job one hundred percent. I saw him administer beatings frequently and with glee. There were among the SS some whom one could call human beings, but I would never count Strippel among them. . . ." Witness Bammbacher describes the defendant as bestial and inhuman, with a reputation among the inmates as being the most infamous. . . . The defendant would walk down the rows of people and kick them in the behind, especially the old, or hit them in the face with his fist or a club.[13]

On May 9, 1940, Strippel married a woman who was as Aryan and Germanic as he. In fact, she even had an SS physician examine her for "racial fitness" and took part in courses given by the German Women's Welfare League in home decorating, folklore, and customs.

After the occupation of France, Strippel—as the SS-Stabscharführer that he was then—transferred his henchman's activities to Natzweiler concentration camp, in Alsace. In June 1942, he moved on to the Jewish death camp of Majdanek, near Lublin. There he was promoted to Untersturmführer.[14]

He had reached his goal of becoming an officer. Now there followed tours of duty at Ravensbrück concentration camp, the labor camp Peenemünde, Vught concentration camp in Holland, the labor camp Drütte, near Braunschweig, and the auxiliary concentration camp Dessauer Ufer, in the Hamburg harbor. Then, as SS-Obersturmführer, he assumed the command of all the Hamburg auxiliary camps belonging to the Neuengamme concentration camp. He had his headquarters at Camp Spaldingstrasse in the inner city of Hamburg, near the central train station and in the immediate vicinity of the concentration camp situated in the school at Bullenhuser Damm.

His career was similar to that of Lagerführer Anton Thumann, who was asked the following by the British prosecutor, Major Wein, during the Curiohaus trial:

> You were unemployed at sixteen. Then you joined the SS, and at twenty you became a professional soldier, as you call it, in the SS. However, according to your own description, throughout your entire career you were nothing more than an executioner, were you not?[15]

After the murder of the twenty children, Strippel seemed to have vanished. On May 31, 1946, British Brigadier General H. Shapcott brought charges against him before the military court in the Hamburg Curiohaus, as well as against Frahm and Speck for the "killing of twenty children at Bullenhuser Damm," but he had to conduct the proceedings without Strippel.

Strippel had gone into hiding, first in Büdelsdorf, near Rendsburg, at the home of an SS buddy, Heinrich Thomsen, later as a farmhand in Hesse. In the fall of 1948, when the SS leaders in West Germany were feeling more secure once again, he presented himself under his real name at the American internment camp in Darmstadt. As a matter of course he received proper documentation and was dismissed.

But on December 13, 1948, at 2:00 p.m., his past met up with him on a street in the center of Frankfurt in the person of an inmate from Buchenwald whom he had subjected to torture by tree-hanging. The man called the police, and Strippel was arrested.

On May 31, 1949, the trial against Strippel was begun in Frankfurt. Strippel was charged with having committed severe injuries in innumerable cases and also with the murder of twenty-one inmates.

These twenty-one—all Jews—were murdered in retaliation for the assassination attempt on Hitler during his speech in the Hofbräukeller in Munich on November 8, 1939. The court accepted Strippel's own description of the mass murder:

> The inmates were ordered by Hauptscharführer Blank to approach the SS-Kommando in about-face. An SS man stood behind every Jew. When the order "move" was given, all the inmates scattered in different directions. As they did, each SS man had to shoot the Jew assigned to him but not before Blank fired the first shot. . . . He, the defendant, did not participate in these shootings, because the whole affair affected him to the depth of his soul.[16]

What happened then was described by inmate Walter Poller in his book *Arztschreiber in Buchenwald:*

> Shortly after ten o'clock Hauptscharführer Strippel called me up on the telephone. His voice sounded harsh and drunk: "Well, do you know where the twenty-one shitheads are?"
> I didn't know for sure how to answer. I had no doubt, of course, as to the fate of the Jews; I also knew that you didn't have to weigh your words when speaking with the Hauptscharführer. But the tone of his voice was so gruesome that I quickly decided to play dumb.
> "No idea, Herr Hauptscharführer," I said.
> Thereupon Strippel screamed like a wild bull into the phone: "Up your ass, that's where they are! Do you hear?!"
> "Yes sir, Herr Hauptscharführer."
> "Go on, then, and write your reports," he said considerably more toned down and stuttering slightly. "Do you need the numbers?"
> "Yes, Herr Hauptscharführer."
> Strippel then dictated to me over the telephone the twenty-one prisoner numbers and the twenty-one names. I went to the files, pulled twenty-one cards, wrote twenty-one death certificates, and wrote twenty-one times as cause of death: —— "Shot while trying to escape." The next day I saw the corpses in the barracks morgue. They had all been shot in the back of the head at close range. The wounds were dreadful, but at least they died instantly.[17]

On June 1, 1949, the court passed its sentence: Strippel was sentenced to "twenty-one life terms for complicity in murder in twenty-one cases committed in Buchenwald Concentration Camp on November 9, 1939." On top of that, he received ten years for inflicting severe bodily injury "in an undetermined number of cases."

He was put in Butzbach prison, where he had it rather good. "Armin, they called him, tall, a typical German," recalls Werner Schütz, a fellow prisoner.

> I knew him for twenty years—from 1949 to his release in 1969. He was errand boy for the prison doctor and had a large room with windows from floor to ceiling. Heinrich Baab, the Gestapo chief of Frankfurt, was his friend. Strippel had a lot of influence in the prison. The members of the infirmary staff were on very friendly terms with him, and they addressed each other with the familiar "Du." He had only done his duty in the concentration camps, he said. "Of course you did kill a few, didn't you," I once said to him. "Of course," he said. Once he also spoke about Bullenhuser Damm.

About this matter Werner Schütz later declared that Strippel had admitted to him that children too had been murdered in Camp Bullenhuser Damm.

Other prisoners report that the group of Nazi criminals in Butzbach would celebrate Hitler's birthday every year on April 20. One of these men was Werner Heyde, known as "the Euthanasia Professor," who after the war and with the knowledge of politicians in Schleswig-Holstein was able to hide under the assumed name of Sawade and work for the municipal offices of the city of Kiel. Strippel would have had double reason to remember April 20. It was the day that the children had been murdered.

But allegedly he knew nothing about this, and on May 10, 1965, he said so for the record to Chief Prosecutor Münzberg, when the latter sat across from him in the office of the Butzbach prison:

> Today is the first time I am hearing about an execution that is said to have taken place in the cellar of Bullenhuser Damm School. I neither received orders for such an execution nor passed on such orders to my subordinates. Where I spent the night of April 20–21, 1945, I can no longer say after twenty years. I assume that I spent it in my room in the Spaldingstrasse camp.

He did dictate a tiny correction, however, since he probably found his own assertion unbelievable:

> When I said that I had heard about the execution in the Bul-
> lenhuser Damm School today only for the first time, I would like
> to have this statement understood as follows: The fact that hang-
> ings had taken place in the cellar of the school, specifically an
> execution by hanging on the night of April 20–21, 1945, these
> are facts I learned about only after the war.

Strippel denounced as a plot against him statements made by the four others who were party to this crime—Trzebinski, Frahm, Jauch, and Dreimann—to the effect that he, Strippel, had been their accomplice.

> The fact that my name was repeatedly mentioned in the Neuen-
> gamme trial and that various of the defendants frequently in-
> criminated me in connection with the hangings of the children,
> this I can only explain by pointing out that each of the defen-
> dants in those proceedings had every conceivable interest in shift-
> ing the blame of the children's murder onto me, since being
> absent I could not defend myself. This is especially true for the
> statements made by defendant Dr. Trzebinski.

Prosecutor Dr. Münzberg accepted Strippel's contention and stayed the pretrial investigation against the SS-Obersturmführer. On June 30, 1967, Münzberg wrote the following in a "Memorandum" that reads like a statement for the defense. There were no longer any witnesses to the mass murder, he wrote. To be sure, the minutes of the Curiohaus trial—with statements made by Trzebinski, Frahm, Jauch, and Dreimann—constitute the main body of proof, but these "can be judged only with the utmost caution." He continued:

> For these statements—at least those concerning the events in the
> cellar of the school—consist exclusively of those made by mem-
> bers of the SS who had been involved in the events and who in
> the meantime had been executed. . . . They also did their best to
> present the facts of the case in the best possible light for them-
> selves and to minimize their own involvement as much as they
> could.[18]

But Münzberg never was able to prove this to be so. On the contrary, when these minutes are compared with the personal notes of Trzebinski, Dreimann, and Pauly, and their various defense counsels, with the numerous minutes of the hearings in the preliminary investigations, with the pleas for clemency, and with the letters of farewell written by the condemned men, it becomes clear that the events surrounding the murder of the children had been described correctly in the trial. Originally, Dreimann and Frahm had obviously agreed during their arrest to put the blame on Trzebinski, who had not yet been apprehended. They declared at first that the latter murdered the children by injecting them with poison. No mention was made of the hangings. But in the cross-examinations these contradictions emerged. Unfortunately, Prosecutor Münzberg did not look for and therefore did not find documents that could have been used for purposes of comparison.

And so he concluded: "Many of the defendants at the time made abundant use of the opportunity to make unjust charges against Strippel."

Münzberg made another mistake. He failed to examine the Magdeburg documents of the Heissmeyer trial. In them he would have found the original records of the experiments on the children and the testimony about the execution order. Münzberg also did not make an effort to interrogate Heissmeyer, who was still living at the time and could have given vital testimony about the experiments on the children and about their death.

However, those were the years of the cold war in West Germany. Justice officials were far more reluctant at that time than they are now to ask justice officials of the East German government for cooperation. And so Dr. Münzberg writes in his "Memorandum" simply this:

According to a report that appeared in *Welt* on July 6, 1966, Dr. Heissmeyer was sentenced in 1966 by a court in the Soviet Zone in Magdeburg to life imprisonment for having conducted TB experiments in Neuengamme concentration camp. . . . One cannot expect to gain any further clarification on the question of the defendant's participation in the children's murder from the documents in the Magdeburg Heissmeyer trial—documents as yet not consulted—because the aforementioned trial concerned itself exclusively with the TB experiments carried out on the children at the time and not with the subsequent killing of these children.

Not true, as we know. For the Magdeburg court did investigate the "subsequent killing of the children" in detail. It would have been worth his while for the prosecutor from Hamburg to have looked at the documents instead of drawing his information from a report in *Welt*.

"In any case," Dr. Münzberg writes in his "Memorandum," "it is certain that the killing of the children, the doctors, and the orderlies was ordered by the authorities in Berlin and that it was up to SS-Standortarzt Dr. Trzebinski to see that it was carried out."

Nothing is less certain. To be sure, Lagerkommandant Max Pauly had claimed in his own defense that the execution order went out from Berlin directly to the Standortarzt and that it fell to him to carry out the murder of both the children and the adults. However, in the Curiohaus trial the British Military Tribunal had already considered this claim as refuted.[19]

And from all other sources—from the Pohl trial in Nuremberg to the great Frankfurt Auschwitz trial—there emerges a chain of command that never excluded the Kommandant of a concentration camp in the case of executions. He was always the central figure.[20]

Whenever an execution was carried out the Lagerführer or the officer next in rank always had to be present. A physician was never allowed to conduct executions but only to establish the death of those murdered. Moreover, it contradicts all SS logic to have entrusted such an important execution to Standortarzt Trzebinski, who was considered a weakling and a coward, in contrast to the hardened Strippel.

To support his assumption, Münzberg points out that Trzebinski had the higher SS service rank. He goes on to say that Trzebinski lied in his claim that "Strippel was authorized to give him (Trzebinski) orders and therefore was also able to give Jauch and Frahm directives in regard to the killing of the children." Münzberg continues:

> On the contrary, Strippel could not tell Trzebinski anything at all. Although Strippel was indeed responsible for the Bullenhuser Damm camp, his power was not so far-reaching as to be able to give orders of any kind—and certainly not orders pertaining to medical matters—to the Standortarzt of the concentration camp, who, moreover, had a higher rank than he, Strippel.

Medical matters? Did the children's murder fall within the category of "medical matters"? This theory of a higher service rank, in any case, contradicts actual practice: doctors had and still have higher rank, even in the German army of today, but they are not allowed to give military orders. Their authority to give orders is restricted to the medical domain only. Executions were military matters not within Dr. Trzebinski's purview. Nevertheless, in his interpretation of the facts of the case, Münzberg comes to this surprising conclusion: "Dr. Trzebinski's assertions, insofar as they place blame on defendant Strippel, are totally refuted."

What is equally astonishing is the "legal appraisal" of the murders. Münzberg ascertains that the children were murdered "for vile reasons" and in order "to cover up another crime"; the deed was executed "insidiously" but not "cruelly"; to be sure, the children were murdered "in a beastly way," which must "fill every normal human being with the utmost revulsion." However, "no extraordinary pain or torture" was inflicted on them.

> The investigations did not prove with the certainty that is demanded of them that the children suffered *unduly* before they died. On the contrary, much can be said for the fact that all the children became unconscious as soon as they received the first injection and were therefore not aware of all that happened to them thereafter. *And so, beyond the destruction of their lives no further harm was done to them; and in particular, they did not have to suffer especially long, either in body or soul.*[21]

Münzberg continues by saying that the doctors and the orderlies were likewise not murdered in a cruel manner:

> The method of the hangings used by Dreimann, that is, to pull their legs up off the floor (as unusual a method as this was), did not inflict upon the victims any agony beyond the destruction of their lives; nor was it inhuman from other points of view. In particular the investigations did not prove that Dreimann's chosen method of execution caused death to occur more slowly than the method used later on, namely, having victims stand on boxes and then knocking these boxes away. Also, the fact that the victims had to undress prior to their execution is neither by itself nor in connection with the pulling away of the legs sufficient to characterize these actions as a form of "cruelty."

Considering Münzberg's way of looking at things, it is not surprising that the prosecutor in no way wanted to seek punishment for the murder of the captured Soviet soldiers. Their killing was "neither insidious nor cruel," for

> all these prisoners had to face the possibility that at any hour they could be liquidated by the SS. As it was, they were taken in a guarded truck to an isolated building in the middle of the night and led down into the cellar four at a time. None of them returned. All these people as they approached death could not possibly have been unsuspecting—as is proven by their desperate attempt to escape.

Yet the simple consideration that at least the first four prisoners went down into the cellar not suspecting anything refutes Münzberg's astonishing assumption. The attempt to escape was made only by the last group of prisoners left on the truck, who in the meantime had become suspicious.

Münzberg, however, outdoes himself in trying to exonerate the Obersturmführer: "But if the Russians . . . had committed a crime for which a non-Russian at that time would also have been punished by death, and if the orders of execution were based on *lawful* death sentences," then it was not murder, because "those who participated in the execution of the sentences had not acted against the law."

According to this legal interpretation, one would no longer be able to convict any Nazi criminals in West Germany for the murder of prisoners. Because, just as in the case with Münzberg, one would always have to "start out from a position most favorable to the accused, namely that the Russians were sentenced to death according to law."

So Münzberg stayed the investigations and justified himself for doing so by declaring that "further evidence about the children's murder . . . could no longer be found," since "all active and passive participants in the events at the school were now dead." Chief Prosecutor Helmut Münzberg had this decision to stay circulated in the prosecutors' offices in Hamburg. His superiors signed it and approved the result of the investigation.

But this was not the end of it. Dr. Münzberg not only drew hasty conclusions from the documents but also neglected the essential duty of a prosecutor, namely, to continue the investigation. It was not true that all the participants were dead. Witnesses from Camp Spaldingstrasse were still alive, as were defense attorneys from the Curiohaus trial, members of the British Tribunal, interrogation officer Major

Freud, and Prosecutor Stewart. Heissmeyer was still alive. So was SS-Unterscharführer Hans Friedrich Petersen, who had driven the children's transport to the Bullenhuser Damm School. And janitor Wilhelm Wede was still alive, whom the SS had given permission to stay in Camp Bullenhuser Damm to take care of heating the school. While the children were being hanged in the cellar and while the doctors, orderlies, and prisoners were dying, Wilhelm Wede was somewhere on the ground floor. He later told a fellow worker that he had slept that night. He should have been asked if he had not perhaps heard shots being fired outside, or the screams of the Russians as the bullets hit them; or if perhaps he had not been present when the bodies were taken away; or if he had not seen Obersturmführer Strippel there.

But no one asked him these questions, because prosecutor Münzberg did not carry out a full investigation. On November 27, 1967, five months after the pretrial investigation was halted, Wilhelm Wede died in Hamburg. Another witness gone.

It seemed as if SS-Obersturmführer Arnold Strippel was being favored as much by fate as by the prosecution. When the Hamburg pretrial investigation of him was halted, the Frankfurt court took up his Buchenwald trial once again. It did so for a reason that the German judiciary would hardly have allowed "ordinary" murderers to claim as a "new fact": it seems one of the witnesses for the prosecution had been labeled in another proceeding as being "generally untrustworthy." Even though this witness had been only a marginal figure in the Frankfurt trial against Strippel and was now just as dead as the witnesses to the children's murder, the West German judiciary granted Strippel a reduction in sentence: in 1967 the ten-year prison sentence for severe bodily injuries "in an undetermined number of cases" was reduced to five years. The twenty-one life terms remained unchanged. The twenty-one dead Jews could not be pleaded away.

But Strippel made another coup: legal proceedings were allowed to resume because Strippel possibly might not have acted as a fanatical Nazi in the murders in the quarry, as the court had consistently assumed until now. At the same time, the court rescinded the arrest order. The SS-Obersturmführer left Butzbach prison on April 21, 1969. He was a free man again. Five months later a new trial against Strippel was begun in Frankfurt. He had in the meantime found work as a clerk with the firm Stempel-Eck, where he kept the books and sent out the bills.

The new trial was a protracted one. Many prisoners who could have testified against Strippel had died. Concentration camp prisoners do not have a long life expectancy.

"The defendant's personality was put in a more positive light as the witnesses for the prosecution softened their statements or withdrew them altogether; a few witnesses even attested to the defendant's humane behavior," Karl Peters, professor of criminal law, ascertained.[22]

After five months the court announced its verdict: It was a fact that on November 9, 1939, Strippel had participated in the shooting of the following twenty-one Jewish prisoners in the quarry of Buchenwald:

Walter Abusch, 17 years old
Herbert Adam, 36 years old
Manfred Adler, 18 years old
Wilhelm Cohn, 24 years old
Herbert Deutsch, 25 years old
Otto Frischmann, 28 years old
Joseph Godel, 32 years old
Arthur Gross, 26 years old
Leo Jablonski, 38 years old
Erich Jacob, 28 years old
Stephan Kende, 51 years old
Theodor Kriesshaber, 55 years old
Julius Levite, 28 years old
Emil Levy, 31 years old
Arthur Maschke, 33 years old
Ernst Meyer, 35 years old
Hermann Rautenberg, 27 years old
Alfred Schafranek, 40 years old
Franz Schneider, 36 years old
Leo Unger, 43 years old
Kurt Wolffberg, 25 years old

But the court claimed that the murderers of the Jews were in fact not the SS who had put the bullets in their heads but Lagerkommandant Karl Koch, who had been dead for some time already. In 1945 his own SS buddies had shot him because he had murdered the personal masseur of SS General Prince zu Waldeck. So now the actual perpetrators were merely "accomplices." And one would have to credit Strippel, after all, with the fact that in 1970 he was "no longer the harsh Rapportführer of Buchenwald, no longer the 'actual accomplice' who should be punished, but a man who had definitely undergone an inward change." The court did not explain, however, how it recognized this inner change.

The court also said on his behalf that Strippel "truly believed that he could get ahead—as all young men earnestly try—by adopting a soldierly demeanor, with the hope of reaching his goal by adhering to a falsely understood sense of obedience." And finally the judges took into consideration that "the administration of justice had become steadily more lenient with the passage of time since the atrocities committed under the Nazi regime."[23]

The murder of Jews was no longer so terrible. And the fact that a person committed such murders to advance his career in the SS did not increase punishment but mitigated it. With this kind of leniency the Frankfurt judges, Seiboldt, Steffgen, and Dr. Zander, punished Strippel for his role as accomplice to murder with six years imprisonment—precisely the same time he had already served in Butzbach prison.

Moreover, Strippel received compensation for his time in prison in the amount of 121,500 marks—seven times more than the amount his concentration camp prisoners would have received as reparations for the same period, had they outlived Strippel. "According to the West German Laws of Compensation, bank robbers and SS torturers are better provided for than former concentration camp victims of the Hitler regime," the former Justice Minister of Hesse, Johannes Strelitz, a member of the Social Democratic Party, commented in resignation.[24]

In 1964 a former inmate, Rudolf Gottschalk, inquired about a criminal prosecution of the children's murderer, and received the following answer from the Hessian Justice Minister at the time, Hemfler:

May I assure you of my own personal sympathy for your bitter fate as a victim of persecution; I can fully understand your indignation over compensation paid to Mr. Strippel for his time in prison. . . . The incongruity between the reparations paid to the victims of the criminal Nazi regime on the one hand and to the perpetrators on the other—perpetrators who after their cases were reopened were either acquitted or had their sentences reduced—this all seems to me so striking that I feel I must point it out to the Federal legislators in some appropriate manner.[25]

Soon after, Rudolf Gottschalk died. He never learned that even this challenge was dismissed by Bonn. "The case of former concentration camp guard Strippel that you cite does not necessitate any change in regulations governing the German compensation laws," the Ministry of Finance wrote in a letter dated May 21, 1973.[26] It went on to say that the German government

> does not intend to make any changes in the regulations—which for all practical purposes have been finalized for some time—governing compensation for immaterial damages due to incarceration of the persecuted victims, not to mention the fact that the compensation due the victims of Nazi persecution had been established conclusively by the German Government's Compensation Law's Final Statute of 1965.

Norbert Gansel, a Socialist Party member of the German Bundestag, was rebuffed in similar manner. He had put these questions to the German Parliament:

> How does the Federal government view the fact that compensation for incarceration in the amount of 150,000 marks was awarded to former SS-Obersturmführer and concentration camp guard Strippel . . . while the victims of the Nazi terror machine received only five marks per day for their loss of freedom? And does the government intend to initiate a change in the Federal Compensation Law so as not to discriminate against these same victims in a way that will not seem so macabre in contrast to the treatment of their torturers?

Nothing of the sort was being considered, Secretary of State Hermsdorf responded during question time in the Bundestag on May 9, 1973.

> Compensation for concentration camp guard Strippel covered only such material damages as loss of pay, social security dues, as well as expenditures connected with his trial,

whereas

> compensation for Nazi victims could have been paid only within the framework of the financial capabilities of the Federal Republic and the states.

And so,

> considering the enormity of the damages and the number of victims, the damages that were incurred by loss of freedom could neither be completely redressed nor fully paid.

In other words, whereas the vast numbers of concentration camp prisoners could receive only a small amount of money, the relatively fewer SS criminals would be generously compensated.

Arnold Strippel bought himself a home in Frankfurt-Kalbach. He had become well-to-do, a member of the middle class who knew how to guard his property and his rights. In fact, when the municipality was planning to establish a public park behind his house, Strippel appeared on April 21, 1978, at a meeting of the community council in Kalbach. One of the participants who was there recalls: "Tall, erect, and sure of himself, this man complained vociferously that the trees that were to be planted would shade his balcony. The Christian Democratic Party took up this request as its own. The trees were planted far away from Strippel's home, and the walks laid in such a way as not to disturb him."

Nine

The SS had these words engraved on their daggers: "My Loyalty Is My Honor." They remained loyal—as did Arnold Strippel—to what they understood to be honor even when mankind believed itself already liberated from them.

When we published the report "Der SS-Arzt und die Kinder" in *Stern* in March 1979, Strippel filed for a temporary restraining order with the court in Frankfurt. He felt his honor had been violated. What he objected to above all was this particular sentence in *Stern* that appeared under his photo: "One of those responsible for the death of the children lives among us: former SS-Obersturmführer Arnold Strippel."

In court he made a statutory declaration, in which he asserted the following:

> The allegations that appeared today in *Stern* No. 11 about my alleged responsibility for the fate of the children murdered in Camp Neuengamme are untrue. At the time in question, Neuengamme concentration camp was under the command of SS-Obersturmführer Pauly. I was in charge of Auxiliary Camp Spaldingstrasse in Hamburg, situated far away. . . . It was only later that I learned of the shocking events concerning the children.

If one reads this statement carefully, one discovers two discrepancies. To be sure, Camp Spaldingstrasse was some thirteen miles from Neuengamme (and Pauly was the Kommandant of Neuengamme), but the children were not "murdered in Camp Neuengamme" but in Camp Bullenhuser Damm—just over a mile from Strippel's Camp Spaldingstrasse. Moreover, he was in charge not only of this auxiliary camp but of all auxiliary camps in the Hamburg region, including the murder site.

However, the third civil chamber of the Frankfurt court disregarded these fallacies, not even giving *Stern* and its authors a hearing, and protected Strippel's honor by issuing a temporary restraining order. On March 9, 1979, *Stern* was prohibited from saying that Strippel "was responsible for the murder of twenty children in Neuengamme concentration camp." And when we did not stop publication of the documentation of the children's murder but printed the minutes of the Curiohaus trial containing Trzebinski's testimony about the hanging of the children, the court imposed a "fine" of 100,000 marks on *Stern*.

April 5, 1979. A lurid scene in Room 122 of the Frankfurt court: Standing there, straight and austere, is a man as broad as a closet, with gray hair on his massive head, wearing thick horn-rimmed glasses: Arnold Strippel. For eleven years he had been a professional henchman in the concentration camps of Europe. Although he was convicted in a court of law of complicity in the murder of twenty-one Jews in Buchenwald, it will never be known for sure how many people he actually tortured to death. His attorney, Dr. Rainer Eggert, speaks of "a cleverly orchestrated execution by the press of a man who cannot defend himself."

The word "execution"—when one looks at Strippel—evokes a taste of blood in the mouth. He denies everything. He was not responsible, and says he never heard a thing. He declares once more: "Each of the auxiliary camps had its own Lagerführer. I was in charge of the Spaldingstrasse camp." What, after all, is a false declaration compared to forty-eight murders?

During one of the recesses his son and bodyguard points to the authors. "There they are. . . !" Strippel turns around. We reflect for a moment: What if it were not 1979 but 1944 and someone said to Strippel, "There they are!" Just as on November 9, 1939, twenty-one Jews were pointed out to him with the words "There they are!"

The court rejects Strippel's plea, contending that "one can no longer give credence to his incomplete declarations." His "participation in the killing of the children" has been made "credible on the basis of the minutes submitted—minutes of the interrogation of the defendants at the time of the Military Tribunal." Even if Strippel had not been convicted of the murder of the children, *Stern* still had the right to call him "one of the perpetrators in the murder of the children."

It should, moreover, also be taken into account that precisely owing to the [then] impending statutory limitations on Nazi atrocities, the press . . . must have the right to report deeds of historical significance, to name names, and to make accusations of complicity. This is especially so when, as here, the person in question (who has said, in his own words, that he was "implicated in the terrible events up to 1945") not only contested his complicity in the events . . . with obviously incomplete statements but elsewhere also admitted it.[1]

(Strippel is said to have "elsewhere admitted" his role in the murder of the children to a former co-prisoner of Butzbach prison.)

In spite of everything, the former SS-Führer makes his appeal to the Supreme Court of Frankfurt: the appeal is dismissed.

Like a traveling salesman dealing in matters of concentration camp murders, Arnold Strippel, former SS-Obersturmführer, made the trip from Frankfurt to Düsseldorf twice a week for five and a half years. From November 26, 1975, to June 30, 1981, he stood there before the court together with thirteen other SS hangmen for murders committed in the Majdanek death camp. Occasionally he also stayed overnight in Düsseldorf. The prosecutor's office had rented a second apartment for him at the expense of the taxpayers.

Strippel looked upon the whole matter very calmly. The accusation against him was comparatively mild. While the others were before the court for the murder of 250,000 inmates,[2] he was answerable for the killing of only forty-two Russian prisoners of war on July 14, 1942. Here, too, Strippel denied everything:

At first the defendant claimed not to have had any knowledge of any inmate killings in the Lublin/Majdanek concentration camp. He had indicated that in his time no inmates had been liquidated, that he knew nothing of any shootings, that he knew the gas chambers only as places for disinfecting clothing, and such.[3]

He even denied his service rank as long as he could.

The defendant at first had denied ever having been Second Schutzhaftlagerführer. In a later interrogation he then said he no longer remembered having been appointed Second Schutzhaftlagerführer. In still another interrogation he admitted that he might possibly have been designated Second

Schutzhaftlagerführer, although he did not feel like one. When presented with documents that he had signed "First Schutzhaftlagerführer" or "Second Schutzhaftlagerführer," the defendant conceded that he may have been substituting for the First Schutzhaftlagerführer but not in cases where serious decisions had to be made.[4]

One day at the trial, in June 1979, eleven Frenchmen are sitting in the gallery. They are the children of murdered Jews. Henri Morgenstern is among them, the cousin of the murdered Jacqueline Morgenstern. He reports:

> A few yards away, his back toward me, sits Arnold Strippel. I recognize him by his profile. My hands become clammy and cold, and I feel a terrible anxiety come over me. It is the horror I feel toward this murderer who hanged my little cousin.

Suddenly the Frenchmen present all jump up and call out: "Nazi murderers!" "No statute of limitations!" "No acquittal for the murderers of our parents!" The judges leave the chamber, as do some of the defendants; but three of them remain, among them, Arnold Strippel. He turns his back on the Frenchmen.

Then Henri Morgenstern begins to speak, in German:

> We are here because we are the children of the victims you have executed. The fact that we are alive today we owe to a miracle. It is unbelievable that there are some of us even left to raise this protest, because almost all Jews were executed.
>
> I see there is a cross here on the wall. Is Germany not a democratic country in which all religions are permitted? Why is there no Star of David next to this cross? If I were arraigned before this court one day, would I have to swear an oath before this cross? It is the truth—a truth you know very well—that Germany today is *judenrein,* or nearly so. This immaculate country, with its wonderful meadows, fields, and forests, has looked upon the murder of Jews also as a matter of keeping itself clean. Before they brought us Jews into the gas chambers, they told us with a smile: "You have to be clean. Take a good shower!"
>
> You want us to be silent so you can continue your kind of justice. But what kind of example of your justice did you show the world when, in this very room, you acquitted four murderers of Majdanek—murderers whose hands were red from the blood

of our brothers and parents! What a disgrace for your system of justice, and what shame the whole world feels for you who dispense justice in such a way! Who are the real victims? These murderers here, or the unfortunate ones they destroyed? We feel shame and so should you!

And that man over there! Look at Strippel, this murderer who doesn't even dare to look me in the face, this coward, this murderer of children! My name is Henri Morgenstern. He hanged my little twelve-year-old cousin Jacqueline Morgenstern, together with nineteen other children in the cellar of the school at Bullenhuser Damm in Hamburg, in 1945.

Look at this murderer and how he hangs his head! What can we learn from him? Has the son learned anything from the father? Yes! He has become a member of a neo-Nazi movement. These people are dangerous, terribly dangerous. I am not speaking here to remind you of a painful past that continues to hurt us. I am speaking here in order to protect my children from the dangers that we have experienced.

Convict these murderers! And do it in such a way that atrocities like these will never again be repeated! If this court defends this murderer, it makes itself into an accomplice. For us that would be scandalous. That's why we cry out here, and will keep on crying out as long as we live: "Condemn the Nazi murderers!" . . .

We will cry out our demands as long as German justice does nothing to win our trust. We don't want revenge; we want justice.

They stand face to face. Strippel is silent. The lawyers call out, "Enough! We've heard all of this before!" Then the police come and clear the chambers. Two demonstrators are injured.

Two years later it becomes evident that Strippel had not been disappointed in placing his trust in the judges. To be sure, he is convicted of aiding in the murder of forty-one inmates; but the gentlemen in their black robes work their magic and conjure up a token sentence of three and a half years in prison—time, as it happens, which the SS-Obersturmführer does not even have to serve. He is, after all, already seventy years old. And there is a long way to go before the verdict is ever to be enforced. The sole restriction on Strippel, then, is that he is not to leave the country—his only punishment for forty-one murders.

When the report about the murder of the twenty children appeared in *Stern*, the relatives of the victims brought charges against Strippel. Dorothéa and Henri Morgenstern, Philippe Kohn, Ans van Staveren (the aunt of Alexander and Eduard Hornemann), Theodora Deutekom (the daughter of orderly Dirk Deutekom), and Alberta Bezem-Hölzel (the daughter of orderly Anton Hölzel)—they all directed Barbara Hüsing, a Hamburg attorney, to initiate murder charges. The prosecution resumed its pretrial investigation of Strippel.

It was at this time that a survivor of another crime appeared on the scene—a sixty-eight-year-old retired woman named Non Verstegen, from Arnheim, Holland. She had been incarcerated in Vught concentration camp for having been an anti-fascist resistance fighter. There she became one of the victims of the "Bunker Drama of Vught." She wrote about this for the record as far back as March, 1946:

> On the evening of January 12, 1944, we had a heated discussion in the sleeping quarters when it was revealed that a German woman prisoner named Jedzini had betrayed former inmates in a letter to the overseer. It was said that these inmates had aided members of the underground. When I put the question to her, she admitted this betrayal. We threatened to cut off her hair if she would do such a thing again. On the very next day already she reported me to the overseer. I was ordered to come in for a hearing. During the lunch break I discussed this new betrayal with my fellow prisoners. We grabbed Jedzini and cut off her hair. She went in and reported us again.
>
> I was taken to Kommandant Grünewald and had to report what had happened. Three times he asked me to give him the names of the others. When I refused, I was punished by being put in solitary confinement in a windowless cell for an indeterminate period, until I would talk. For fifty hours I had to stand in this empty, unheated, dripping wet cell. They took my coat away from me.
>
> Jedzini was so terrified of the consequences of having informed on me that she tried to escape during the night. As she fled she was shot by a guard and a week later died of her injuries in the hospital.
>
> On the evening of my arrest, almost all of the women of Block 23 B, where these events had taken place, went to the

guard's room to give in their numbers. By doing so they wanted to show that they had been in agreement with the hair cutting. This was interpreted as "mutiny," and that Saturday evening at 6:00 all the undersigned were brought in two groups to the prison barracks. When the first group of forty-nine women was put in a small single cell, I was included. The second group followed, and as many as possible were shoved into our cell. Kommandant Grünewald, in the presence of his assistants and Schutzhaftlagerführer Strippel, personally jammed in the last ones, so as to get in as many as possible. We later counted seventy-four persons in one cell. The remaining seventeen, who just could not be pressed in, were put in a cell similar to ours.

In our cell it was so crowded that we were unable to move. There was hardly any air. It took us several hours to open a small casement window that was stuck. By this time a number of the women were already unconscious, and more became so during the course of the night. What made the situation steadily worse was the total darkness in the cell, our raging thirst, and later the sudden fit of insanity of one of the women, who started to bite those around her. We took off our clothes and licked the condensed water dripping off the ceiling. Later we noticed we were getting skin burns from standing against the walls, and also burns on our lips because the freshly painted walls and ceiling were giving off nitric acid. When the door was finally opened at 7:30 a.m. thirty-four women were lying on top of each other in a pile in the middle of the cell. Forty others were leaning against the walls and against each other. We later learned that ten of the women had died. Many others were ill for a long time thereafter, and some of these died later on as a result of that night. For many others still, the ordeal of that night was probably a factor in their subsequent death in the camp, so that the actual number of victims cannot be known for sure.

Non Verstegen, who today is seriously ill and cannot leave her house, also directed Attorney Barbara Hüsing to initiate charges against Strippel. She declared, "I saw how Strippel shoved women into the cell with his own hands."

Attorney Hüsing made a startling discovery: Back in July, 1967, the Dutch prosecutor had sent material implicating Strippel and others to the Central Office in Ludwigsburg—6,000 pages of documents. In July and August 1968, prosecutors in Ludwigsburg passed on these documents in two separate dispatches to the prosecutor's office in Frankenthal, Rheinland-Pfalz, since a pretrial investigation was being carried out there against Benno Hüttig, the last Kommandant of Vught concentration camp. At that time, Frankenthal received material that also implicated Strippel.

Eleven years later, then, in April 1979, Attorney Hüsing sought to find out what had happened to this Dutch material. She was told that in these Frankenthal documents there was partially untranslated evidence in Dutch. It could not be determined if it also contained material that might possibly serve as evidence against Strippel. To find out, obviously one would have to know Dutch.

So for eleven years this evidence concerning ten counts of murder lay untouched in the prosecutor's office in Frankenthal because no Dutch translator could be found. How, then, did matters stand in the case of evidence in Polish or Serbian or Russian?

Attorney Hüsing asked the Minister of Justice of Rheinland-Pfalz to look into the matter and to consider the criminal consequences, since obstruction of justice in office—as, for example, neglecting to deal with criminal charges—is a crime punishable by six months to five years imprisonment.[5]

Minister of Justice Otto Theissen, however, informed her upon brief consideration that there was "no cause for initiating a pretrial investigation."[6]

Ten

Many people make it easy for themselves and speak of blood-thirsty beasts, of devils, of born criminals, or of subhuman beings when they mean concentration camp guards. But Strippel is no devil, Dreimann no beast, Trzebinski not subhuman, Pauly no born criminal.

As unobtrusively as most of these people blended back into everyday life after the end of the Nazi era—becoming clerks, police officials, doctors, or businessmen, respected by their neighbors—they were just as unobtrusive before the time of their crimes. They were ordinary people.

From his death cell Wilhelm Dreimann writes to his wife:

Well, Mutti, if fate would turn and bring us back together again, I would wish for only one thing—to live for you all. It's what I wanted to do even in the last years of our separation. My life until now has been nothing but work and struggle. I've never had many happy hours.[1]

The unhappy life that Wilhelm Dreimann spoke about began already with his unhappy childhood. "His parents raised him strictly, and being a son of a laborer, he was conditioned early on to hard work," Dreimann's wife writes in her plea for clemency.

It was difficult for him to get ahead in his job as a woodworker, so in 1939 he signed up for service in the regional police. Against his wishes he was inducted into the SS at the beginning of the war, and as far as I know he tried time and again to leave it and to return to police service. However, his request was never passed on or considered.[2]

This is not quite true, since in 1939 only volunteers were taken into the SS. But pressing need and fear of joblessness made many people carry out every order from above. His wife continues:

> He was a man with a strong sense of duty, on whom it was impressed even as a child to be obedient. He knew nothing beyond doing his duty as a soldier, but this very eagerness to serve and to do his duty, and the prohibition against speaking about official matters, hardened him and made him dissatisfied. And thus he may have carried out his orders to the letter, for there was no way he could act against them as a soldier.[3]

This attitude is as typical for the average man as the "nonpolitical" attitude: "My husband was never active politically; he was popular with everyone in our village. . . . He was a caring family man."[4]

Dreimann even claimed to be inwardly and totally at odds with the severe policies of the Nazis, with regard to both the persecution of the Jews and the tortures carried out in the concentration camps. But the regime gave the orders, and one had to obey. Thus he writes in a letter to his wife from prison that he did not beat Kurt Schumacher, a Social Democratic Party politician:

> Dr. Schumacher was brought to Neuengamme after July 20, 1944. I don't recall when he was released. Please ask him how I treated him when he was brought in. . . . I could never understand at the time why old and frail people should be robbed of their freedom in such a manner, and I said as much to them, although perhaps covertly, since I was not able to speak out openly then against the directives of the regime. . . . I don't need to justify myself any longer. I know that my testimony will vindicate me in the eyes of the world and of humanity.[5]

It was not only fear of punishment that moved almost all of the concentration camp criminals to profess their good consciences before the world and before humanity. It was also a compulsion to seek justification for themselves. They had been trained to be obedient, to be subservient, to suppress their moral qualms. They had been nothing but obedient, so why was that so wrong? They had never criticized the state, because it was hammered into them that to do so was one of the worst crimes they could commit.

Max Pauly, the son of an ironmonger from Wesselburen, in

Schleswig-Holstein, was also one of those indoctrinated into this kind of obedience to the state. A middle-class mentality, combined with ever-increasing economic difficulties, moved him to join the S.A., Hitler's original shock troops, as early as 1928. He was a ruffian and a brawler, who was always afraid of economic ruination. His attempts to join the civil service finally landed him a position in the lower ranks of the SS. "I participated all along in the growth of the SS in Schleswig-Holstein," he writes in an autobiographical statement. His education and his knowledge of history always remained at the very bottom of the scale.

While in prison he writes to his son, Hans-Werner:

> Whatever may happen, my dear boy, believe firmly in the innocence of your father, and never be shaken from your faith in me. As a soldier I did my duty for my fatherland until the end. I administered the now infamous Neuengamme camp for two and a half years with the best of intentions, always trying to ease the life of the inmates as much as was possible. I am only glad that you saw the camp yourself and so can form your own opinion.[6]

Pauly does not understand that the judges in the British court hold him responsible for actions ordered by his superiors: "Because I was the Lagerkommandant they hold me responsible for everything that happened in Neuengamme," he writes in another letter:

> I am made to bear the brunt of directives and orders of my superiors, including executions. And even things that were perpetrated by Thumann, Dreimann, or other block leaders they now charge me with. I will just have to bear the consequences as a German. . . . For your peace of mind I want to emphasize today that I am not aware of any fault of mine, and that I always acted in the interests of the prisoners, doing my duty to the very end.[7]

He feels drawn to bear responsibility "as a German" but not as a perpetrator. Nor does he admit to having "perpetrated" anything of the sort that he claims the others did. All he did was to carry out orders, including executions, in the interest of the prisoners. On the other hand, he complains in the same letter about "these mad policies of Hitler and his criminals," which are of "incalculable consequences for the German people." And so Max Pauly was another humble underling whom one could train to commit crime because he lacked altogether the capacity to criticize the state.

Dr. Alfred Trzebinski came from a very different background from Pauly. He was the son of a high school teacher from Jotruschin, in the Rawitsch district of Poland, which the Nazis called Orlahöh. He studied in Breslau and Greifswald and was supported by the alumni of his fraternity. In turn he expressed a submissive gratitude toward them, while at the same time feeling disdain and condescension toward all nonacademics. His professional qualifications were modest. He scorned medical science, believing instead in Providence, ghosts, the horoscope, laying-on of hands, mesmerism, and iridiagnosis. In his handwritten diary, entitled "I," composed in his death cell, he describes a visit made to a healer:

> A doctor colleague of mine from Hamburg—like me a wearer of the SS uniform and for that reason most likely in the same situation as I am now—took me to see Emiel Nietz, the iridiagnostician. A man of immense reputation, he was sought for consultation by the most highly placed and important people. His professional judgments were definitive. When Hermann Göring was to have an operation of the maxillary sinus and the surgeons could not agree among themselves, Emiel Nietz, the healer without a medical degree or title, made the decision to operate! And the surgeons operated. When Nietz was summoned to Heinrich Himmler, he could read from his eyes that Himmler had two birthmarks below the left knee. Himmler pulled up his trousers and looked at these marks in amazement, never having noticed them before. . . .[8]

Trzebinski believed his illusions to be real. He once said that he had seen "the man in black, alive and real. . . ."

> I had fled Breslau because the all too intense fraternity life distracted me from my real goal in life, my medical studies. I thought that I could make up in a small university town on the Baltic what I had left undone in Breslau. However, as soon as I arrived there, I was eagerly taken in by a student corps associated with my own. I realized soon enough that the students here knew much more about drinking than in Breslau. Indeed, due to a lack of other diversions they were paying homage to Bacchus with incessant offerings. . . .
>
> Suddenly, as if swept by a windstorm, the door to my room flies open and bangs against the wall, knocking off chunks of

plaster, and in walks an incredibly dried up, tall fellow clothed in black from head to toe in old-fashioned garb, stockings pulled over bony calves, rumpled hair framing a gaunt, yellow face with a sharp nose and dark, piercing eyes. He slowly walks toward me, lifts up his right arm, and points his finger at me as he approaches the foot of my bed. I let out a scream of terror, totally devoid of any human sound, and thrashed about in my bed. The door slammed shut with a crash so that the walls shook, and the spectre vanished.[9]

Trzebinski's dreams of black-clad figures, symbolizing death, foreshadowed the SS, who took up this unsuccessful country doctor from Mühlberg, Saxony, into its black ranks and sent him to the sites of their blackest crimes—to Lublin, Auschwitz, and Neuengamme.

Such illusions, typical of an alcoholic, repeated themselves and were interpreted by Trzebinski as somehow connected to the supernatural. Once he thought an old woman wearing a kerchief was standing at the foot of his bed, pointing toward "something that seemed to lie far beyond the walls of the room."[10] Another time the wall opened up and a "figure diffused in light sat on a golden chair . . . while on both sides of this golden throne figures in black stood poised in two long straight rows near my bed."[11]

He had recurrent dreams about his life being somehow interwoven with that of Marie Antoinette because they had the same horoscope. He found allusions to this everywhere: In his prison cell there was a magazine picture of her pasted on the wall. He was given her biography from the prison library. She, too, he noted,

> had been condemned because she represented a regime no longer in power, and in her case too no consideration was given to whether or not such representatives were personally guilty. . . . She, too, had behaved in an exemplary fashion to the very end, and only concern for her children caused her grief. . . .[12]

Until they were executed the twenty children caused him the same kind of grief, he noted. And to give them morphine injections before the hangings had been a humane act, he felt. His whole life was marked by self-pity. Time and again he sought recognition—even before the British Military Tribunal. Instead of loving human beings, he took refuge in love of animals: "Such an almost morbid love of animals (of which I admit I am not ashamed) does not happen by chance. . . ."[13]

Trzebinski could not stand to see animal blood. He would cry over a slaughtered rabbit and was constantly afraid in the Neuengamme concentration camp that his pet cat Muschi would somehow get hurt: "Be careful of the electric fence and all the bad dogs out there!" he would warn her.[14]

Before the British came, "in April of that fateful year of 1945, in the final month of German freedom," Trzebinski was concerned about the future of his dear Muschi and her new litter of four:

> After my departure, who would be around to care for this happy, devoted, and unsuspecting creature? Perhaps a rough kick by a soldier's boot might once and for all have made her lose her faith and trust in man. So I raised my pistol. Muschi noticed nothing and was dead on the spot. Her kittens, still on the threshold of consciousness, I drowned in a barrel of water.[15]

By way of contrast, note the entry on his participation in the execution of human beings:

> I left the bodies hanging for half an hour, then examined them to determine if they were dead, and had them removed. . . . But I cannot understand why doctors who fulfill the unquestionably necessary task of determining death are charged with this as a crime, even in the case of an illegal execution. After all, a physician, by performing this kind of examination, prevents any chance of a person being buried while still alive.[16]

This is the way specialists talk. One is a specialist in administration, including the administration of concentration camps. The other is a specialist in meting out punishment, including punishment with the leather whip. The third is a specialist in determining death, including death by hanging. And if it was all ordered by higher-ups, it cannot be considered unlawful; it must be within the law because it emanates from the state.

And what about today? "What was lawful then cannot be unlawful today," according to Hans Filbinger, a former West German Prime Minister. This may not be a commonly held view, but it is the view of a radical minority. Were we to have a new fascism today, could it again make use of people like Strippel, Dreimann, Pauly, and Trzebinski? They surely still exist today—these people who knuckle under, who are loyal to the state to the point of injustice, who are loners, who love animals more than human beings, who are full of hatred toward those who are exposed to them as enemies of their state: Jews, gypsies, Poles, leftists, communists.

People like Strippel, Dreimann, Pauly, and Trzebinski are not the architects of fascism, not its financiers, not its beneficiaries. But they are the ones who would again be needed to support a new fascism. For they are the ones who guard, beat, execute, and, at their best, administer a merciful injection of morphine beforehand.

Eleven

One would have thought that after Germany's liberation from the Nazis the people of Hamburg would have made Bullenhuser Damm School into a memorial to the dead children and their companions. But after housing the library of the Naval Weather Observatory, the building once again became a school, three years after the end of the war. Any concern that such a place of murder might produce fear in six-year-old children was not recorded in the minutes of the teachers' conferences.

To be sure, under the heading "Preparatory Work" one does find something said about renouncing this terrible past:

> Primers and readers for the elementary grades will be cleansed of passages and pictures that would detract from an education conducive to fostering peace. . . . We want to try with all our hearts to educate our dearly-tried German youth to become honest human beings who love and practice justice and truth, who go out into life conscious of their responsibility, considerate of their fellow men, industrious and peace-loving.

Yet not a single word is said about how precisely this school, like no other on earth, could show young people the difference between responsible and irresponsible human beings. Instead, only this much is mentioned:

> Concerning the Problem of Bullenhuser Damm: A request was made by parents to Senator Landahl at the Socialist Party district meeting in the Bille Brewery to use the Bullenhuser Damm building as a school once again. The primary reason being the poor roads on Bullenhuser Island.[1]
>
> The question was thereupon taken up in the parents' council. Parents' meeting on this topic is to be held at a later time.

Priority needs would be, first, new chairs (which will be difficult to deliver in the necessary number).

Then several additional problems are discussed—problems such as heating fuel, number of students, a janitor, and, most important, the question of coeducation. Additional minutes record the following: "We will agree to the transfer to Bullenhuser Damm on condition that the traditions of the Brackdamm Boys School be continued in the new school building and that the piano purchased by the boys' school can be taken along as well."[2]

On August 25, 1948, the teaching staff inspected the school building at Bullenhuser Damm: "Benches are still needed for five classes," they noted in the minutes. Then the rooms are carefully assigned—from workroom to science room. Still no word about the cellar where the murders took place.

On September 20, 1948, the children move back into the old building. The school is decorated with flowers, parents come, as do important school officials. There are speeches. A sports festival is held. Not a word about the dead children.

Have they been forgotten? Do they want to forget them? Two years later, on August 23, 1950, a single sentence appears in the minutes: "Mr. Behr reads a letter from the VVN [Association of the Victims of the Nazi Regime] and suggests that mention be made in class of the memorial service referred to in the letter." That is all.

And yet people such as Pauly, Heissmeyer, Trzebinski, and Himmler did not attain their goal of having this crime and its perpetrators sink into oblivion. The comrades in suffering—the other inmates of Neuengamme—kept the memory of the tortured children alive in their hearts. Every year on the day of the murder they went to the school at Bullenhuser Damm and placed flowers there.

It was not easy for them to gain entry. The small cellar room where the children were hanged was crammed full of junk. In addition, almost all the former prisoners belonged to the VVN, and in Adenauer's Germany this organization was considered "a front for the communists" and was actually banned in the State of Hamburg.

There was a time when it was dangerous to admit to remembering the children. In March of 1956 ten-year-old Monika Bringmann wrote a letter to the editor of the Children's Page of the *Norddeutsche Echo* in Kiel: "These crimes must never happen again!" She described the murder of the children of Bullenhuser Damm and the Curiohaus Trial. In conclusion she wrote: "I myself cannot believe that human beings treated children in this way. Such crimes must never happen again, and all children who read the Children's Page should write in and express their opinion."

The Criminal Police in Winsen an der Luhe considered Monika Bringmann's letter a punishable defamation of the state and wanted to question the child. But her father prevented this from happening. Monika was the daughter of the same Fritz Bringmann who, as an inmate in Neuengamme, had refused to carry out the SS order to kill Soviet prisoners. And he was raising his children to follow the same moral principles.

Writer Willi Bredel describes another case in his book *Unter Türmen und Masten*.[3] A teacher at Bullenhuser Damm School had called upon his colleagues to speak to the children in class about the murderous actions of the SS in the cellar of the school. "Most of the teachers, however, decided not to touch upon this secret." So the teacher took it upon himself to tell the pupils that their school had once been a children's concentration camp. As punishment for this he was denounced to the educational authorities and later even held in detention for a time.

There was even an attempt to connect Willy Brandt, the Social Democratic Chancellor of West Germany, in some way to the murder of the children. As the only chancellor who had actively resisted the Nazis, Brandt was hated by many people in Germany. Attacks on him turned to blind hatred when he concluded the East-West pact with the Soviet Union and Poland and when he went down on his knees at the memorial for the fallen victims of fascism in Warsaw, on December 7, 1970.

On March 19, 1970, Gidon Rynar, a businessman from Bonn, wrote to the police saying that the murder of the children in Hamburg had been committed by a certain SS-Rottenführer Frahm. He, Rynar, wanted to have them check to see if this same Frahm could possibly be Chancellor Willy Brandt, who, as everyone knows, was the illegitimate child of a Mrs. Frahm from Lübeck. Dr. Sarembe, a Hamburg prosecutor, began a pretrial investigation of Willy Brandt. She found that it was not Willy Brandt who had committed the murder but Johann Frahm, who in the meantime had been executed. She ordered the legal proceedings[4] against Brandt to be stopped in 1971 because "all means of investigation had been exhausted." Then she also sent a copy of her ruling as a precautionary measure to the "Central Office" in Ludwigsburg—just in case Willy Brandt should ever come under suspicion again.

Time and again the former concentration camp prisoners asked the Hamburg Senate and school officials to make the murder site into a memorial room and to provide it with a plaque.[5] In the meantime, an international organization of former prisoners of Neuengamme had been established, called Amicale Internationale de Neuengamme.

Pressure from abroad definitely helped. On January 30, 1963— on the thirtieth anniversary of the Nazi dictatorship—a memorial plaque was affixed. To be sure, it was not "on" the school building, as the former inmates had always hoped and as the senator had promised, but all the same it was *in* the school—in the stairwell of the school, removed from public view. There were flowers, wreaths, and an address by the Minister of Education.

On the simple tablet one reads:

> This is where twenty foreign children and four adult companions were murdered on the night of April 20–21, 1945, a few days before the end of the war, by lackeys of the Nazi regime. Let us remember the victims with love. Let us learn to respect man and all human life.

(No mention is made of the twenty-four Russian soldiers who were hanged with the children.)

That year and every year thereafter a small memorial service was held on April 20 at the entrance of the school. The Senate sent a wreath, the school officials a speaker. The survivors of Neuengamme brought flowers. But every year there were fewer survivors. And every year the story of the children's death slipped further into the past. It seemed like an event from long ago, from a past in which no one lived any longer. Not the victims, not their families, not those who did the deed.

It was simply by chance that the names of the children were preserved. A Danish physician, Dr. Henry Meyer, had brought them with him out of Neuengamme. He had been a prisoner there himself for a year and a half and had been freed in the rescue operation of the Swedish Red Cross. In the final days before his departure, he worked as a doctor in the "Scandinavian Camp" of Neuengamme.

After his return on May 6, 1945, he wrote a "Report for the Danish Red Cross," which appears in the book by Swedish Professor Rundberg entitled *Rapport fra Neuengamme*.[6] In it Henry Meyer describes the medical experiments on inmates, mentions the TB experiments of Heissmeyer, and gives the names of the children.

It is possible that he obtained the list of names from another Neuengamme inmate, but this can no longer be clarified. Dr. Meyer, who had worked for many years at the district hospital in Apenrade, died in the early 1960s.

This list of names, however, did not help very much when we started our search for the relatives of the children, for at the end of their regime the Nazis had destroyed all concentration camp records.

But we finally did find the family of the two brothers, Alexander and Eduard Hornemann. With the aid of a Dutch journalist, Albert Eikenaar, we discovered in the Rijksinstitut voor Oorlogsdocumentatie in Amsterdam the reference that they came from Eindhoven. We found the house at 29 Staringstraat, where the Hornemanns had lived until the end of 1942, when their house was requisitioned by the Germans and given to a security official named Vorberg. The house at 49 Gagelstraat also still exists—that is where the Philips bus stopped on August 20, 1943, and brought Elisabeth "Bets" Hornemann and her two boys to the Vught concentration camp. If she had gone with her sister Ans to Old Pastor Vonk's hiding place in Aarle-Rixtel, they may all have been spared death in the camps. "Tante Ans" still lives in Utrecht. She had learned of her sister Bets' death right after the end of the war, from fellow inmates from Auschwitz who had returned after liberation. But no one knew what had happened to the two children after they were taken away during roll call in front of their barracks in Auschwitz that September morning in 1944. "Tante Ans" had always kept the hope alive that they might have disappeared somewhere in Russia and would come back to her some day. She wept bitterly and could not sleep for many nights when she heard that the children were dead. And yet it was better to know, as she put it, than to live with thirty years' of uncertainty.

Philippe Kohn said the same thing. He was Georges Kohn's brother. We found him with the help of Paris attorney Serge Klarsfeld, who published a collection of documents containing the names of the deported Jews of France.[7] On the list of Convoy No. 79 there appeared the names of the Kohn family. But only Philippe Kohn was still alive. He was fifty-three years old and lived in a suburb of Paris.

After he and his sister Rose-Marie had jumped off the deportation train, they were kept hidden by the stationmaster in St. Quentin until the Americans liberated them. Then they had both returned to Paris.

There is a photo that shows Rose-Marie and Philippe with a group of others who had fled the train; they were all celebrating May 8, 1945—the date that marked the end of German fascism, a day when the world could breathe freely once again. Philippe and Rose-Marie Kohn look sad on this photo: they did not know anything then about the fate of their parents and their brother and sister, Georges and Antoinette.

A few weeks later their father, Armand Kohn, returned from Buchenwald very ill. And then they learned that their mother and sister Antoinette had starved to death in Bergen-Belsen. They searched for Georges everywhere among those returning; they even found some eyewitnesses from Auschwitz; but then they reached a dead end. Finally, Georges André Kohn was declared dead, and the French government awarded him the hero's title, "Mort pour la France"—"he died for France." Until they died Armand Kohn and his daughter Rose-Marie (who succumbed to cancer at a young age) heard nothing more about Georges. Philippe wept when we brought him the news: "My poor little brother!"

Among the 75,721 names of deported Jews we also found the name of Jacqueline Morgenstern. Together with her father Karl (born 10/6/03) and her mother Suzanne (2/19/07), she had been transported on June 20, 1944, with Convoy No. 74 from the Bourget-Drancy station to Auschwitz. It had been a large transport, numbering 1,388 people. Of this number 49 men and 108 women came back alive. The three Morgensterns were not among them.

But there were some relatives left in Paris, living in the old Jewish quarter of Belleville: Dorothéa Morgenstern, an aunt of Jacqueline, and her son, Henri Morgenstern, a dentist. They had been keeping a record of Jacqueline's fate under the German occupation.

Here is an excerpt from Dorothéa Morgenstern's account:

> Jacqueline's father and my husband were brothers. Charles and Leopold Morgenstern had a large beauty salon in the rue Beaurepaire #8 on the Place de la Republique. When they got out of military service in 1940 they reopened their business. There were many Germans among their customers. In 1941 an Aryan administrator by the name of Cornilland was put in

charge. All Jewish shops were given such administrators. Cornilland had our store signed over to him by a notary public in Orléans and gave each brother 25,000 francs. I did not want to sign, but Suzanne said: "What do you think is better, to go to Drancy or to sign?" So I said, "If that's the case, then I'll sign."

In 1942 they were looking for us. Poldi had received a pass certifying that he was working—making jackets for Stalingrad, fur jackets for the Germans. So he got a scrap of paper giving him permission to stay. But Charles did not have such a permit, so he hid for a time in the Eighth Arondissement, where Suzanne's sister had a small flat. However, there was no way he could live there for very long; nor did he have anything to eat. So Suzanne went to see this Cornilland and asked him for help: "Mr. Cornilland, the shop is now yours, and we are in such a desperate situation. Maybe you can help us. Can you get my husband over to the other side?" Cornilland said he could, that he had an acquaintance over there: "I'll get your husband across, and from there he can go on to Marseilles."

Once Charles was in Marseilles, his wife and daughter joined him there. Suzanne had borrowed a French identity card and glued her photo on it. She gave away everything she owned. That was in September of 1943.

I never saw them again—not Suzanne, Charles, or Jacqueline. They lived in a small room. Suzanne found work as a steno-typist, and Charles worked at whatever came his way. Jacqueline went to school without any problems. After all she was already a twelve-year-old girl by then.

In the meantime they were looking for us again. We lived then at 31 rue de Belleville. On October 18, 1943, at 11:00 p.m., there was banging on the door: "Police!" We did not open. For five minutes we did not move. Then the police shouted again: "We know you're in there. If you don't open up, we'll break down the door." So we said, "Break down the door? They know we're here?" So we opened the door.

There were two men standing outside, one with a gun in his hand. We raised our hands—my husband, Henri, and I. My little boy Jackie was in bed with a fever. I fainted, and Henri began to vomit all over the place from nervousness. He was nine years old then. Then Henri called out, "What are we, some kind of murderers or thieves, that you break in on us like this in the middle of the night?"

When I came to and could speak again, I said: "I'm pregnant, and my child is ill. Why don't you leave my family be? Tell them you didn't find us at home." But they refused. So Papa took his knapsack, and Henri was also dressed and ready to go. He had a little bag on his back.

In the meantime the neighbors had called a doctor. He gave me a shot and told the police that if they took me along I would surely die on the way. My husband then told them: "Take me but let my wife and children stay!" He pulled the ring off his finger, took out his watch and chain, and gave them all to me. So they let us stay behind and took him along, saying: "We'll be back tomorrow."

Very early the next morning we had already left the house. We went to a "dispensaire" where the Organisation OSE[8] was located. They placed the children, and I did not know where they were and how they were doing until the liberation. Every month a woman doctor, Dr. Breton, went to see how the children were doing, and all she told me was, "Your children are alive, they're alive." I found out only after the liberation that they had been kept hidden in the little village of La Chapelle du Bois de Feu in Normandy, near Evreux. They came back in November 1945.

In the meantime I gave birth to my daughter in secret—as "Madame X," because I was in the hospital anonymously. My daughter was therefore called Françoise Marie Anni X. Then a woman doctor took me to her home. She was a very, very fine lady, this Madame Chatelain, and she kept me with her for six months. During this time I got a letter from Marseilles, from Suzanne. She wrote: "Dear Dora, we read every letter from you with great sadness, our eyes full of tears. But I know that you are brave in the hope that you will see your husband and children one day soon. You see, we too have been together again for the past three months, and it seems to me as if we had never left each other. Charles had many troubles while we were separated, and so did I. But all that is now forgotten, and we hope that it will be the same for you one day. Even in one's own misfortune one sees others who are more unfortunate still."

But they themselves were soon to become the most unfortunate of all, when they were denounced and arrested in Marseilles. Jacqueline was home alone doing her homework. The French police came and asked her: "Do you know where your mother is?" She told them that she was working and also where she was working. They took the child along, and she had to show them where Suzanne was working. They took Suzanne with them and told her to get her things packed. Then they went to where Charles was working, but he had been warned and had run off.

When he got to the house across the street and observed how Suzanne and Jacqueline were brought to the car, his daughter cried out: "There's my Daddy!" And so Charles was also arrested. All three of them perished. Suzanne in Auschwitz, Charles in Dachau, and Jacqueline at Bullenhuser Damm.

But we learned of this only long after the liberation. I wanted to get back into my flat at that time, but it was occupied by a neighbor, and only after taking legal action did I manage to have it returned to me in 1946. In the meantime I had been living in a hotel room no bigger than my kitchen is today. All four of us slept on the floor. When my children returned, they were all infested with lice, but I thanked God that I had them back alive.

One day a post card came from Poldi, from Dachau. It was postmarked May 8, 1945. He wrote in German, "I'll be home soon." Whenever there was a knock on the door the children would call out, "That's Daddy." But it was not. Instead, a man came one day when I was not at home and told my neighbor that Poldi had died soon after being liberated because he was so weak. My neighbor did not take down this man's name, and I never heard from him again. Only a death certificate came one day from Germany.

Later we tried to get our shop back. Cornilland was able to hire two lawyers; I had to receive free legal assistance. The lawyers insisted that the shop had not been taken away forcibly but that we sold it voluntarily. As proof they produced the letter Suzanne wrote to Cornilland when they were all in Marseilles: "Dear Mr. Cornilland, my husband got here safely. He is already with my relatives, and I thank you very much for the service you have done for us. With greetings and thanks. Suzanne Morgenstern."

This letter was read in court. I was present. The judge emphasized that a person to whom one writes such a note of thanks could not have been an enemy, but only a friend. He let Cornilland keep the shop.

If I think back to those difficult times, most of all I remember Madame Chatelain, who knew my children and had such compassion for us. She fed me well, cared for me, gave me a room, and provided for my child. May God reward such people with good things for all that they did for us.

Much has happened since the report about the children's murder at Bullenhuser Damm was first published. Thirteen children have been positively identified, and the search continues for the other seven. In many cases valuable information has been provided by surviving relatives or townspeople. Dorothéa Morgenstern, the aunt of the murdered Jacqueline Morgenstern, probably spoke for all of the survivors when she wrote to the author: "As a result of your efforts, the dead children are no longer quite so dead."

On April 20, 1979, the relatives of the murdered children stood at the murder site for the first time. Instead of the usual handful who would come each year to observe this anniversary at Bullenhuser Damm School, on this day there were over 2,000 people. They had brought flowers, covering the walls of the school with blossoms.

On the same day, the surviving family members founded an association called Children of Bullenhuser Damm, to keep alive the memory of the murdered children in Hamburg, to promote antifascist education in the city's schools, and to combat neofascism.

And so the promise made to the twenty children by the inmates of Neuengamme and inscribed on the ribbons of the floral wreaths becomes a reality: "Dear children, we have not forgotten you."

These are their names:

Alexander Hornemann, 8 years old, from Holland
Marek Steinbaum, 10 years old, from Poland
Eduard Hornemann, 12 years old, from Holland
Marek James, 6 years old, from Poland
W. Junglieb, 12 years old, from Yugoslavia
Roman Witónski, 7 years old, from Poland
R. Zeller, 12 years old, from Poland
Sergio de Simone, 7 years old, from Italy
Georges André Kohn, 12 years old, from France
E. Reichenbaum, 10 years old, from Poland

Jacqueline Morgenstern, 12 years old, from France
Surcis Goldinger, 11 years old, from Poland
Lelka Birnbaum, 12 years old, from Poland
Eleonora Witónska, 5 years old, from Poland
Ruchla Zylberberg, 10 years old, from Poland
H. Wassermann, 8 years old, from Poland
Lola Kligermann, 8 years old, from Poland
Rywka Herszberg, 7 years old, from Poland
Blumel Mekler, 11 years old, from Poland
Mania Altman, 5 years old, from Poland

GLOSSARY

Blockführer	An SS n.c.o. in charge of one or more blocks of prisoners; reported to the Rapportführer
SS-Brigadeführer	Brigadier General
Gauleiter	The highest ranking Nazi official below the Central Government; responsible for a Gau, or region
Hauptscharführer	Master Sergeant
Hauptsturmführer	Captain
Kommandoführer	An SS n.c.o. in charge of prisoners' units, often organized as work details
Lagerältester	An inmate responsible for order and discipline in the barracks and on the camp grounds
Lagerarzt	Camp Doctor
Lagerführer	Assistant to the Commandant of a concentration camp; responsible to the Lagerkommandant for maintaining discipline among inmates
Lagerkommandant	Chief officer of a concentration camp responsible for the entire camp
NSDAP	Nationalsozialistische Deutsche Arbeiter Partei (National Socialist German Workers' Party)—the official title of the Nazi Party
Obergruppenführer	Lieutenant General
SS-Oberscharführer	Platoon Sergeant
SS-Obersturmbannführer	Lieutenant Colonel
Obersturmführer	First Lieutenant
Rapportführer	An SS n.c.o. in a concentration camp responsible for taking roll calls and performing other administrative duties
Reichsführer-SS	Himmler's personal title as head of the SS
Reichsstatthalter	The Reich governor of a Land or a Gau
SS-Rottenführer	Corporal
Schutzhaftlagerführer	An assistant commandant of a concentration camp

SS (Schutzstaffel)	The strong-arm force of the Nazi Party
Sonderkommando	Teams of concentration camp inmates used in the gasing and cremation of other inmates
SS-Sonderkommando	A special detachment of the SS used for specific police and political duties
SS-Stabscharführer	Staff-Sergeant Major
Standortarzt	Senior Physician
Standortkommandant	Senior commandant
SS-Sturmbannführer	Major
Stützpunktleiter	Assistant to the commandant of a concentration camp
SS-Unterscharführer	Sergeant
Untersturmführer	Second Lieutenant
Waffen-SS	The militarized combat forces of the SS

NOTES

Chapter 1

1. Protocol of the Nuremberg "Doctors' Trial," 1947, pp. 404–05.
2. Alexander Mitscherlich and Fred Mielke, *Medizin ohne Menschlichkeit* (Frankfurt, 1978), pp. 69–70.
3. Dr. Josef Mengele, from Günzberg, went into hiding after the war, first in Argentina; there he married the widow of his brother, co-owner of Mengele and Sons, a large factory for farm machinery in Günzberg. For twenty years he lived as a millionaire in a villa near Asunçion under the protection of the President of Paraguay, General Antonio Stroessner. Since early in the summer of 1979 Mengele has once more disappeared.
4. Robert Neumann, *Hitler: Aufstieg und Untergang des III. Reiches* (Munich, 1961), pp. 178–79.
5. Ebbo Demant, *Auschwitz-direkt von der Rampe weg* (Reinbeck, 1979), p. 57.
6. *Przeglad Lekarski*, I (Cracow, 1967), pp. 3–4. In this report Mrs. Piekut-Warszawska describes in detail the experiments by Mengele with Jewish twins. Also published in the anthology *Auschwitz*, II, 3 (International Auschwitz Committee), 1–11.

Chapter 2

1. *Przeglad Lekarski*, I (Cracow, 1967), pp. 3–4.
2. *Przeglad Lekarski*, I (Cracow, 1965); Auschwitz, II, 3, pp. 18–19.
3. Rudolf Höss, *Kommandant in Auschwitz*, dtv documents 2908, p. 109. SS-Obersturmbannführer Rudolf Höss was Kommandant of Auschwitz from May 4, 1940, to November 10, 1943. During this time he built the largest factory for the destruction of human beings in history. On March 11, 1946, he was arrested by the British Military Police near Flensburg and on May 25, 1946, extradited to Poland. During his time in the Cracow prison he wrote a comprehensive report on his life as a henchman. On April 2, 1947, the Supreme People's Court in Warsaw sentenced him to death. Höss was hanged on the gallows of Auschwitz on April 16, 1947.
4. See the report by Hanna Hofmann-Fischel in Yad Vashem, the Israel Holocaust Museum and Documentation Center in Jerusalem. Selections have been published by Inge Deutschkron under the title . . . *denn ihrer war die Hölle: Kinder in Ghettos und Lagern* (Cologne, 1965), p. 54.
5. Deutschkron, . . . *denn ihrer war die Hölle*, pp. 63–65. Jehuda Bacon, who survived Birkenau, gave the following testimony on October 30, 1964, at the Auschwitz Trial in Frankfurt. His description of the gas chamber and the technical aspects of the gasing process is essentially the same as the one Lagerkommandant Höss gives of his machinery of destruction, which he calls

a "discovery": "We had now discovered the gas and also the procedure for using it. I had always dreaded the mass shootings, the shootings of women and children. I had had enough of the executions of hostages, of the mass executions ordered by the Reich Security Service or the Reich Security Main Office. I was now relieved that we would all be spared these bloodbaths, that the victims could be spared until the last moment."

At the gasings that he conducted he himself was often inclined to weep. Höss recalls: "Once two little children were so engrossed in their play that they did not want to be torn away at all from it by their mother. Even the Jews of the Sonderkommando did not want to take up the children. I will never forget the pleading look of the mother, begging for mercy though she certainly knew what was to happen. The people in the chamber were beginning to get restless—I had to act. Everyone looked at me—I gave the acting subordinate a nod, and he took the children, who were resisting strongly, into his arms and brought them to the gas chamber together with the mother, whose weeping would break one's heart. I wanted to disappear off the face of the earth out of compassion—but I was not allowed to show the slightest feeling." (Höss, *Kommandant in Auschwitz*, p. 132.)

6. On November 13, 1952, the firm J. A. Topf and Sons, which had been relocated after the war, from Erfurt to Wiesbaden, applied to the government patent office for a patent to protect the design of Crematorium II, which had been tested at Birkenau. Patent No. 851,731 was for "a method used for the cremation of corpses, cadavers, and parts thereof by means of recurrently heated air."

7. After January 17, 1945, Auschwitz was cleared in batches. As a result many thousands of inmates lost their lives through hunger and thirst, shootings, and freezing to death in open container cars. On January 27 the first patrols of the Red Army liberated the camp.

8. Interrogation of Heissmeyer, March 10, 1964, pp. 197–99 of the court records, Magdeburg.

9. Otto Prokop and Ehrenfried Stelzer, "Die Menschenexperimente des Dr. med. Heissmeyer," *Zeitschrift Kriminalistik und forensische Wissenschaften*, 3 (1970), p. 92.

10. Interrogation of Heissmeyer, September 8, 1964, pp. 227–28 of the court records.

11. Ibid.

12. Interrogation of Heissmeyer, March 11, 1964, p. 108 of the court records.

Chapter 3

1. Protocol 01/166–117/37 in Yad Vashem, Jerusalem.

2. Jan Everaert. He lives today in Ghent.

3. *Prozess Neuengamme*, I (Hamburg, 1969), p. 188.

4. Prokop and Stelzer, "Die Menschenexperimente . . .," p. 103.

5. Dirk Deutekom, a typographer, was born on December 1, 1895. He was arrested in July 1941, with a group of Dutch resistance fighters in Amsterdam. They had armed themselves in an effort to prevent the deportations of the Jews. In Buchenwald concentration camp Deutekom was trained as an orderly. On June 6, 1944, he was transported to Neuengamme and worked there in the sickbay.

Driver Anton Hölzel, born May 7, 1909, was a member of a communist group in the underground and active in the struggle against fascism. As a waiter in a coffee house in Den Haag he was able to gather messages and transmit them. On September 11, 1941, he also was arrested and transported, first to Buchenwald and then to Neuengamme. Together with Dirk Deutekom he volunteered to take care of the "Heissmeyer children."

6. Interrogation of Czekallá, December 17, 1945, by Captain A. W. Freud; transcript in possession of the author.

7. Hans Klein, since the war Professor of Forensic Medicine at Heidelberg University. He informs the author by letter: "The lymph nodes that were brought here in 1945 were examined like all other organs or tissue parts sent to a histology lab. The serial numbering of individual lymph nodes could indicate that an experiment was involved. I learned about the experiment only from the documentation of the later Heissmeyer trial."

Heissmeyer testified about Klein (who worked as a pathologist at the SS sanatorium in Hohenlychen) at a hearing on March 30, 1964: "Certain preparations were sent to Hohenlychen. There a pathologist who had also been with me at the Neuengamme camp examined them." (p. 252 of the court records on Heissmeyer.)

Professor Klein contests this in a letter to the author of May 18, 1979: "A visit with Heissmeyer in Neuengamme did not take place, nor did a joint plan for experimentation, either there or in Hohenlychen. Heissmeyer treated me for my tuberculosis at Hohenlychen, so I spoke with him frequently about the current state of TB research as far as my expertise allowed me. To what extent the experiments were influenced by these conversations I can hardly determine. I did not say or do any more at Hohenlychen than any other pathologist would have said or done."

8. *Prozess Neuengamme*, III, p. 346.

9. H. R. Trevor-Roper, *The Last Days of Hitler* (New York, 1947), p. 116.

10. Report from the High Command of the Wehrmacht, April 21, 1945.

11. Reitlinger, *Die SS Tragödie einer deutschen Epoche* (Vienna, 1957), p. 427.

12. Felix Kersten, *Totenkopf und Treue* (Hamburg, 1952). The letter of safe conduct read as follows: "To whom it may concern. It is requested that Senior Medical Officer Felix Kersten and the gentleman accompanying him be allowed to cross the border without presentation of identity papers. Schellenberg, SS-Brigadeführer, Major General of the Waffen-SS and Police."

13. Ibid.

14. Gerhard Rundberg, *Rapport fra Neuengamme* (Copenhagen, 1945), pp. 63–64.

15. Odd Nansen, *Fra dag til dag* (Oslo, 1947), 3, pp. 274–76.

16. Jørgen H. Barfød, *Helvede har mange Navne* (Copenhagen, 1969), p. 336.

17. Rundberg, *Rapport fra Neuengamme*, pp. 34–35.

18. Carl Krebs, *Pigtråd*, XVII, p. 45.

19. Rundberg, *Rapport fra Neuengamme*, pp. 60–61.

20. Barfød, *Helvede har mange Navne*, p. 338.

21. Ibid., p. 339.

Chapter 4

1. Wilhelm Dreimann, SS-Unterscharführer, Rapportführer of Neuengamme concentration camp. Heinrich Wiehagen, SS-Unterscharführer in Neuengamme. Adolf Speck, Kommandoführer in Neuengamme.

2. This and subsequent quotations by Trzebinski are taken from *Prozess Neuengamme,* a collection of documents compiled by former inmates of Neuengamme (III, pp. 347–350).

3. Barfød, *Helvede har mange Navne,* pp. 239–240.

4. The doctor was Professor Florence.

5. *Prozess Neuengamme,* I, pp. 247–52.

Chapter 5

1. Federation of Former Neuengamme Camp Inmates *(Lagergemeinschaft Neuengamme), So ging es zu Ende* (Hamburg, 1960).

2. Rudi Goguel, *Cap Arcona* (Frankfurt, n.d.), p. 26.

3. Ibid., p. 27.

4. Ibid., p. 57.

5. Ibid., pp. 60–61.

6. Heinrich Mehringer, "Cap Arcona," *Neuengamme-Informationen,* XVIII (Hamburg, 1962).

7. Goguel, *Cap Arcona,* pp. 65–66.

8. Federation of Former Neuengamme Camp Inmates, *So ging es zu Ende,* p. 66.

Chapter 6

1. British Protocol, JAG 145, II, Day 18, p. 87. Located in the Public Record Office, London.

2. Federation of Former Neuengamme Camp Inmates, *So ging es zu Ende,* p. 68.

3. Record of the hearings, transcript in possession of the author.

4. Ibid.

5. Ibid.

6. British Protocol of the Curiohaus Trial, JAG 145, I, Day 1, p. 14. Located in the Public Record Office, London.

7. In 1978 Fritz Bringmann published a documentary report, *Der Kindermord von Bullenhuser Damm* (Frankfurt: Röderberg Verlag).

8. Adlershorst is located near Danzig, where Pauly had been Kommandant of the Stutthof concentration camp.

9. Original letter by Pauly, in possession of the author.

10. Original notes by Trzebinski, in possession of the author.

11. Original letter of May 1, 1946, in possession of the author.

12. SS-Obergruppenführer Oswald Pohl was head of the SS Economic and Administrative Office. He was in charge of all concentration camps. Pohl was sentenced to death in 1947 in one of the Nuremberg trials and was executed in June 1951 in Landsberg. Prior to this he had returned to the Catholic Church and received the Apostolic Blessing from the Pope by telegraph. Pohl made the following extenuating statement about Heissmeyer's experiments: "Heissmeyer, Department Head in the Medical Institute at Hohenlychen, received permission from Himmler to carry out TB experiments. I sent him to Gluecks, who put the necessary human subjects at his disposal. These were about ten children, probably from Auschwitz, who did not have parents. The experiments took place in Neuengamme. I later saw a paper about these experiments that was meant for Himmler. But it was so technical that I was not able to understand it." (Document NO-065 Pohl Trial,

Institut für Zeitgeschichte, Munich.) Pohl's superior was SS-Obergruppenführer August Heissmeyer, the uncle of SS-Doctor Kurt Heissmeyer of
Hohenlychen.

13. British Protocol, JAG 145, II, Day 14, p. 43.

14. Ibid, Day 15, pp. 4, 5.

15. Ibid, pp. 29, 30.

16. Plea by Dr. Curt Wessig, April 17, 1946, at the Curiohaus Trial,
Hamburg, p. 17.

17. Plea by Wessig, p. 21.

18. British Protocol, JAG 145, V, Day 37, pp. 23, 24.

19. Ibid., Day 38, pp. 51, 52.

20. Copy in possession of the author.

21. Plea for clemency by Mrs. Lisbeth Dreimann, addressed to the Supreme Military Tribunal in Hamburg, May 8, 1946; copy in possession of the
author.

22. Letter of farewell by Trzebinski, in possession of the author.

Chapter 7

1. Cited from court records of the Prosecutor General, East Germany.

2. At the "Doctors' Trial" of the American Military Tribunal in Nuremberg, August 20, 1947, Karl Gebhardt was sentenced to death and was later
executed.

3. Original letter by A. Kutschera-Aichbergen, July 27, 1964, in possession of the author.

4. Lord Russell of Liverpool, *Geissel der Menschheit (Scourge of Humanity;*
Berlin, 1956)*: "When in April the Allied troops were fast approaching
Neuengamme, SS-General Pohl, at the request of Dr. Heissmeyer, gave the
order to take the children to the camp at Bullenhuser Damm and to execute
them there, so as to do away with all evidence of the experiments." (pp. 197–
98.)

5. Prokop and Stelzer, "Die Menschenexperimente des Dr. med. Heissmeyer."

6. Letter by Otto Prokop to the author, November 22, 1978.

7. Kirst became ill with TB after the liberation and had to undergo
surgery.

8. Prokop and Stelzer, "Die Menschenexperimente. . . ," pp. 75, 76, 91,
92, 94, 102, 103.

Chapter 8

1. Strippel was not SS-Hauptsturmführer (Captain) but an SS-
Obersturmführer (First Lieutenant).

2. What a farce the so-called denazification program actually was has
been reported by the former Nazi mayor of Hamburg, Carl Vincent Krog-
mann, in his book *Es ging um Deutschlands Zukunft,* which although filled with
Nazi propaganda was published in 1976 by the Druffel Verlag without any
objections being raised. On page 12 he describes the denazification hearings
of his case, which took place on August 14, 1948, in Bielefeld: "Shortly before
the start of these hearings the public prosecutor came to my defense attorney
greatly disturbed, saying he had just received directives from Hamburg
charging him to ask for a prison sentence for me. He said he could not

reconcile it with his conscience to follow these directives. My attorney assured him not to trouble himself, that he had spoken with the chief judge—a prison term was out of the question. Despite the directives, the prosecutor then delivered a speech for the defense that was all I could have hoped for. The judgment bore out that I had been a decent fellow."

3. According to Delegate Dr. Menzel, 1960.

4. A. Baring, *Aussenpolitik in Adenauers Kanzlerdemokratie* (Munich, 1971), I, p. 152.

5. Charles W. Thayer, *Die unruhigen Deutschen,* p. 252.

6. Falko Kruse, "NS-Prozesse und Restauration," *Kritische Justiz,* 2 (1978).

7. Reinhard M. Strecker, *Dr. Hans Globke* (Hamburg, 1961).

8. A. Baring, *Aussenpolitik. . . ,* p. 92. The newspaper is said to have received a total sum of 265,000 marks.

9. *Spiegel,* 45 (1968), p. 42.

10. Publication of the Ministry of Defense, I, September 1, 1956 (Bonn).

11. Personal papers of Arnold Strippel, Document Center, Berlin.

12. Verdict of the Frankfurt Regional Court, June 1, 1949.

13. Verdict of the Frankfurt Regional Court, 1949, pp. 11–14.

14. Untersturmführer corresponds to the rank of a lieutenant in the German army, according to the "General Dispensation" made by the Minister of Defense, September 1, 1956.

15. British Protocol, JAG 145, III, Day 21, p. 76.

16. Verdict of the Frankfurt Regional Court, June 1949, p. 6.

17. Walter Poller, *Arztschreiber in Buchenwald* (Hamburg, 1947), p. 136.

18. This and subsequent citations are taken from Memorandum 147 (June 30, 1967) of Chief Prosecutor Münzberg, found in the Arnold Strippel papers, Hamburg State Archives.

19. Explanation by Chief Justice Stirling prior to the verdict. British Protocol, JAG 145, V, Day 38, p. 51.

20. See the verdict in the Frankfurt Auschwitz Trial, pp. 44–46: ",IV Ranks, Chain of Command." See also the explanation by SS-Standartenführer Gerhard Maurer, Amtschef D II in the WVHA of the SS, July 11, 1947, in the Pohl Trial in Nuremberg, Document ZS 567-P2 (Institut für Zeitgeschichte, Munich).

21. Emphasis added. In a conversation with the author on February 23, 1979, Chief Prosecutor Dr. Helmut Münzberg regretted having formulated this sentence. He was sure he would never again write another sentence like this one.

22. Karl Peters, *Fehlerquellen im Strafprozess,* II, p. 337 (Karlsruhe, 1972).

23. Verdict of the Frankfurt Regional Court, File no. 19/8, Ks 6/49, pp. 53–54.

24. Quoted from *Die Glocke vom Ettersberg,* 51 (Frankfurt, 1973).

25. Letter, in possession of the author, from the Minister of Justice of Hesse to the Federation of Former Buchenwald Camp Inmates, December 29, 1972.

26. Letter in possession of the author.

Chapter 9

1. Verdict of the Frankfurt Regional Court, April 5, 1979, File No. 2/30111/79.

2. The International Military Tribunal in Nuremberg determined that

altogether some 1,500,000 people were murdered by the Germans in Majdanek.

3. Indictment against Hermann Hackmann, File No. 8 Ks 1/75, p. 115.

4. Ibid., p. 114.

5. Section 258a of the Penal Code. In less severe cases imprisonment for up to three years or a fine. The attempt to obstruct justice is also punishable.

6. Six months later it turned out that the Minister of Justice had lied. There most certainly was cause for initiating a pretrial investigation against the prosecutor's office. Just as postwar Germany had solved other such embarrassing interludes in the cover-up of Nazi murders, so also did it solve this one: the Minister of Justice had to step down. And the colleagues of Prosecutor Beisswenger (who had been singled out as the only one responsible for suppressing the Dutch material for eleven years) initiated a pretrial investigation against him. But this was soon halted, because obstruction of justice in office is punishable only if it can be proven that the offender acted with intent. And Beisswenger's colleagues did not want to go after this proof.

Chapter 10

1. Letter of Wilhelm Dreimann, May 31, 1946, to his wife. Copy in possession of the author. In the same letter Dreimann also writes, however, that his wife should not believe a former inmate (B. from Drieburg) who had called on her: "B. was not imprisoned in Neuengamme for political reasons but because he was a professional criminal, and his personal papers may well reveal that he had already lost his teeth before he was brought to Neuengamme."

2. Plea for clemency, by Mrs. Dreimann to the British Military Court, May 8, 1946.

3. Ibid.

4. Ibid.

5. Undated letter of Willy Dreimann to his wife, in possession of the author.

6. Letter of Max Pauly to his son, Hans-Werner Pauly, May 1, 1946.

7. Letter of Max Pauly to his sister-in-law, Leni Hilgenstock, April 14–15, 1946.

8. Alfred Trzebinski, "Ich," unpublished manuscript in possession of the author.

9. Ibid., pp. 25–29.

10. Ibid., p. 17.

11. Ibid., pp. 22–23.

12. Ibid., p. 4.

13. Ibid., p. 65.

14. Ibid., p. 78.

15. Ibid., pp. 79–80.

16. Undated handwritten notation by Dr. Trzebinski during the Curiohaus Trial, 1946; in possession of the author.

Chapter 11

1. Bullenhusen is an island in the center of Hamburg located between Bille and Bille Canal. Because of the destruction of the bridges during the war, the island character of this part of the city became especially prominent.

2. Minutes of the Teachers' Meetings, 1948. Found in the archives of Bullenhuser Damm School.

3. Willi Bredel, *Unter Türmen und Masten* (East Berlin, 1968), pp. 422–440.

4. Injunction 147 Js 15/70, by the Prosecutor's Office, Hamburg; copy in possession of the author.

5. Thus, for example, Fritz Bringmann writes in a letter of September 17, 1959, to the Hamburg Minister of Education, Heinrich Landahl: "I would request that the rooms in Bullenhuser Damm School in which the unfortunate children and their companions became victims of the dehumanized SS be restored in a worthy manner; that a plaque be placed there in their honor; and that the rooms be decorated on memorial days." Heinrich Landahl writes in response on September 19, 1959: "At the beginning of this year I ordered that preparations be made for a memorial plaque. I have before me a number of possible inscriptions, but I am not yet satisfied with them."

6. Rundberg, *Rapport fra Neuengamme,* p. 108.

7. Serge Klarsfeld, *Le Memorial de la déportation des juifs de France* (Paris, 1978).

8. *Oeuvre de secours aux enfants*—a Jewish children's relief organization. Members of this organization were in close contact with the French Resistance and tried to place children of arrested and deported Jews, under false names, with Christian families.

INDEX

175